Good Housekeeping

Drop a Dress Size

Anita Bean BSc RNutr

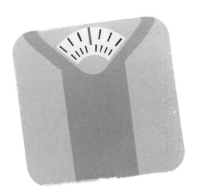

Contents

Everyone talks about calories as if they are something contained in food. But what exactly are they? Calories are simply a measurement of energy, just as a kilogram is a measurement of weight and a mile is a measurement of distance.

If you take in more calories than your body uses, you'll gain weight as the body stores fat. If you use more calories than you take in, you'll lose weight.

Your calorie requirement depends on your genetic make-up, age, weight, body composition and activity level. It will differ from one day to the next, depending on how active you are, and also change as you grow older. As a rough guide, it's about 2,000 calories a day for an average woman and 2,500 calories for an average man. For a more accurate estimate of the number of calories you use during daily life and when exercising, go to http://nutritiondata.self.com/tools/calories-burned. Enter your gender, age, weight, height, lifestyle and daily exercise undertaken.

If you eat 3,500 more calories than you need, they will be stored and add 450g/0.5kg (1lb) to your weight. On the other hand, burn 3,500 more calories than you eat and you'll lose 450g/0.5kg (1lb). This isn't as daunting as it seems. By eating a little less and being more active, you can achieve a daily calorie deficit of 500; for example, you could cut out a packet of crisps and a glass of wine to save 300 calories, and walk an extra 40 minutes to burn 200 calories. Over a week, this would result in a calorie deficit of 3,500 and a weight loss of 450g/0.5kg (1lb). Losing 450g/0.5kg (1lb) a week amounts to 7kg (15½lb) in 14 weeks, or 26kg (4 stone 1lb) in a year.

Experts agree that a healthy and effective rate of weight loss is between 450g/0.5kg (1lb) and 1kg (2¼lb) per week. Don't try to lose more than this, otherwise you risk fatigue, excessive muscle loss and a significant drop in your metabolic rate, making weight loss harder. Drastically cutting calories can lead to insatiable hunger, making you more likely to binge on high-calorie foods and pile the weight back on. Worse, your body can end up hoarding, instead of burning, fat. Your body goes into survival mode and the rate at which you burn energy slows down. Your body adapts to survive on a lower calorie intake, which means that when you stop dieting, you're likely to put the weight back on.

The key is to find a plan that you can comfortably live with, rather than attempting to lose weight periodically with strict diets that are hard to maintain. This book will help you to drop a dress size in six weeks with ease, just in time for that special event.

HOW TO USE THIS BOOK...

First, complete the Diet Decoder Quiz on the next page to find out what kind of eater you are. This will help you avoid the dieting pitfalls. Now, discover how to change your eating habits. You are then ready to work through the chapters that follow, covering eating at home and at work, in restaurants and when buying takeaways, as well as how to shop wisely and how to have fun at parties without affecting your weight-loss goals. The Drop a Dress Size way provides a six-week plan, giving you weekday meal planners that you will find at the end of each chapter. There are recipes in the chapters themselves as well as at the back of the book. At weekends, use the portion sizes and substitution knowledge from the book to eat wisely whether you're eating out at a restaurant or enjoying Sunday lunch at home – allow yourself a little flexibility without going overboard. Each chapter also includes exercise workouts (and Chapter 5 is devoted to improving your fitness), as it's an essential part of your Drop a Dress Size plan.

The exercise programmes in this book are intended for people in good health – if you have a medical condition or are pregnant, or have any other health concerns, always consult your doctor before starting out.

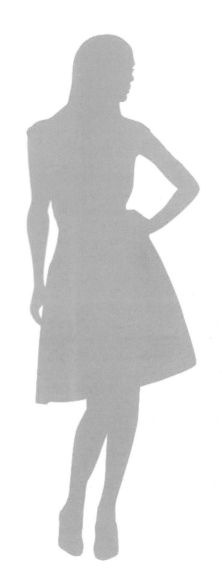

DIET DECODER QUIZ

By determining your personal diet pitfalls, you'll be primed to transform your bad habits into weight-loss success, one small and healthy change at a time. This quick quiz will help you do just that. Circle your answers and tally your results on page 8.

1. When I'm hungry, fast food is an easy option; I often stop and grab something – chips, a burger or perhaps a doughnut.
A. Rarely (0 points)
B. Sometimes (1 point)
C. Often (2 points)
D. Always (3 points)

2. Although I never think about crisps and never buy them, if they're in front of me (such as at a party), I'll automatically snack on them.
A. Rarely (0 points)
B. Sometimes (1 point)
C. Often (2 points)
D. Always (3 points)

3. I'm usually not hungry in the morning, so I tend to leave the house without eating breakfast.
A. Rarely (0 points)
B. Sometimes (1 point)
C. Often (2 points)
D. Always (3 points)

4. I drink 'energy' or 'health' drinks.
A. Rarely (0 points)
B. Sometimes (1 point)
C. Often (2 points)
D. Always (3 points)

5. I drink juice, fizzy drinks or other sugary drinks a few times every day.
A. Rarely (0 points)
B. Sometimes (1 point)
C. Often (2 points)
D. Always (3 points)

6. When I am upset, I can eat a whole pizza (or a packet of biscuits or a carton of ice cream) in one sitting and still want more.
A. Rarely (0 points)
B. Sometimes (1 point)
C. Often (2 points)
D. Always (3 points)

7. While cooking or preparing food, I'll have so many tastes that I'm not really hungry by the time I sit down to eat the meal.
A. Rarely (0 points)
B. Sometimes (1 point)
C. Often (2 points)
D. Always (3 points)

8. My hunger is often sudden and urgent, and, if I eat a large quantity of food, I feel guilty afterwards.
A. Rarely (0 points)
B. Sometimes (1 point)
C. Often (2 points)
D. Always (3 points)

9. Chips are my favourite vegetable.
A. Rarely (0 points)
B. Sometimes (1 point)
C. Often (2 points)
D. Always (3 points)

10. On very busy days, I may eat just once or twice a day.
A. Rarely (0 points)
B. Sometimes (1 point)
C. Often (2 points)
D. Always (3 points)

11. I often nibble on the foods my family/friends don't finish, even when I'm full.
A. Rarely (0 points)
B. Sometimes (1 point)
C. Often (2 points)
D. Always (3 points)

12. Low-fat cereal/snack bars and sugar-free sweets are staples in my diet.
A. Rarely (0 points)
B. Sometimes (1 point)
C. Often (2 points)
D. Always (3 points)

13. A bad day at work or a family argument can trigger a binge.
A. Rarely (0 points)
B. Sometimes (1 point)
C. Often (2 points)
D. Always (3 points)

14. After a stressful day, food provides a welcome distraction from my anxious feelings.
A. Rarely (0 points)
B. Sometimes (1 point)
C. Often (2 points)
D. Always (3 points)

15. I have takeaway a few times a week.
A. Rarely (0 points)
B. Sometimes (1 point)
C. Often (2 points)
D. Always (3 points)

16. I have at least two beers, glasses of wine, or other alcoholic drinks four or more times a week.
A. Rarely (0 points)
B. Sometimes (1 point)
C. Often (2 points)
D. Always (3 points)

17. I have several cups of coffee or tea with sugar and/or cream or milk every day.
A. Rarely (0 points)
B. Sometimes (1 point)
C. Often (2 points)
D. Always (3 points)

18. While watching TV or a film, I reach for snacks whether I'm hungry or not.
A. Rarely (0 points)
B. Sometimes (1 point)
C. Often (2 points)
D. Always (3 points)

19. At a certain time of day, I find myself ravenous and searching for something to quiet my growling stomach.
A. Rarely (0 points)
B. Sometimes (1 point)
C. Often (2 points)
D. Always (3 points)

20. I'm never sure where or when I'll have a real meal so I tend to eat on the go.
A. Rarely (0 points)
B. Sometimes (1 point)
C. Often (2 points)
D. Always (3 points)

ADD IT UP!

Add points from questions 1, 9, 12 and 15 for your
JUNK FOOD JUNKIE SCORE:

_____ + _____ + _____ + _____ = _____
TOTAL

Add points from questions 2, 7, 11 and 18 for your
MINDLESS MUNCHER SCORE:

_____ + _____ + _____ + _____ = _____
TOTAL

Add points from questions 3, 9, 10 and 20 for your
MEAL-SKIPPER SCORE:

_____ + _____ + _____ + _____ = _____
TOTAL

Add points from questions 6, 8, 13 and 14 for your
EMOTIONAL EATER SCORE:

_____ + _____ + _____ + _____ = _____
TOTAL

Add points from questions 4, 5, 16 and 17 for your
LIQUID CALORIE LOVER SCORE:

_____ + _____ + _____ + _____ = _____

You may find that you indulge in more than one (or even all five) of the behaviours indicated opposite. That's OK. If you have a score higher than six on any of them, just be sure to pay extra attention to the tips targeted at that habit. Throughout the book, the strategies have been tagged to identify the ones that will help you overcome your particular diet pitfalls.

Emotional eaters use food for more than fuel – it also serves as a friend and a comfort. Feelings such as sadness, loneliness, anger or frustration cause these eaters to turn to food for escape.

Junk food junkies fill up on nutrient-poor (empty-calorie) foods. Fast foods, sugary snacks, salty snacks and high-fat fare are the norm; vegetables, fruits, whole grains and other healthy foods are less frequent choices.

Liquid calorie lovers unwittingly load their diet with extra calories from drinks. Fizzy drinks, milkshakes, coffees, cocktails, smoothies, energy drinks and others spell trouble because of their calorific bottom line.

Meal skippers tend to have unbalanced eating patterns and often wait too long between meals. As a result, their meals are not planned or thought out, but rather are last-minute choices made wherever and whenever hunger takes over. They often end up making poor diet choices and cave in on cravings because they're so famished.

Mindless munchers are all-day grazers and unconscious eaters who put food in their mouths out of habit or boredom, regardless of hunger. They'll eat in front of the TV or automatically snack at a party, for example, paying little attention to their hunger cues. When mindless munchers start to track what they consume, they're often surprised at how much they eat during the course of a day.

Remember, transforming just one or two of your daily diet habits can result in pounds lost and a slimmer, trimmer you – in just a few weeks!

The highest total scores on the opposite page represent your principal eating behaviours or habits

To get you started, here are our top tips for slimming down and keeping the pounds off. Make these strategies your mantra, and you will drop that weight. Stick them on your wall, computer, dashboard – wherever you'll see them – to keep you motivated.

1 Believe you can do it

You've already taken the first step by picking up this book. But if your dieting will wavers along the way, don't give up. Think about what's important in your life, such as your family, your job or your home. Now place yourself and your weight-loss goals and health at the top of that list. And don't forget to acknowledge your successes, no matter how small. You avoided that chocolate bar from the vending machine today? Worth a secret inner high five at least! Dropped your first 1.4kg (3lb)? Surely justification for that new lipstick you've had your eye on.

2 Make the most of your calories

By selecting empty-calorie foods, you're spending a lot for something that offers very little – like some insanely expensive, very trendy shoes that give you blisters and are difficult to walk in. They might be fun to wear on occasions, but most of the time you'll want to wear something stylish and comfortable. If you're economising on calories to lose weight, it makes sense to pack a lot of nutrition into what you eat. A food that's loaded with fibre, vitamins and minerals but also low in calories is a nutritional bargain – it's a nutrient-dense food. On the other hand, foods such as fizzy drinks and sweets will load you with lots of calories and are low in vitamins and minerals, making them low-nutrient, calorie-dense foods. Such foods are often called 'empty-calorie' foods, but describing them as empty of nutrients would be more accurate. And remember, nutrient-dense foods will fill you up for far longer than calorie-dense foods.

This doesn't mean that chips, burgers, sweets and other less stellar choices are diet no-nos. The truth is that no food or drink is so high in calories, fat or sugar that including it on occasions in a diet that is healthy overall is going to sabotage your weight loss. Just be sure to keep your total calorie intake within the recommended limits (page 12), and you'll still drop a dress size. Here's what to look for:

- **Fruits and vegetables** Rich in nutrients and low in calories, fruit and veg are a dieter's best friend. There's no such thing as a bad fruit or vegetable, but the more variety you eat, the better.

- **Low-fat dairy** These versions of milk, cheese, yogurt, cottage cheese and so on, are packed with nutrition and have fewer calories than the regular versions.

- **Lean proteins** Lean meat, poultry and fish, as well as vegetarian choices such as beans and tofu, will help you feel full and stay that way.

- **Whole grains** Select fibre-rich, wholegrain foods such as oatmeal, wholemeal bread and wholegrain rice instead of refined grains such as white bread, white pasta and white rice.

- **Healthy fats** Choose olive and rapeseed oils, avocados, nuts and nut butters, seeds and olives – but remember, a little goes a long, long way. A drizzle of olive oil on your salad, a small handful of nuts with your cereal, or a few slices of avocado on your sandwich all add satiety and flavour.

3 Get the facts

Be your own food detective, online and off, and you'll not only uncover surprises about what's hiding in your food but you'll also set yourself up for success. Check out In the Supermarket (Chapter 4) for tips on how to fill your trolley with the right foods, and Eating Out (Chapter 3) for the insider info you need to make the best choices, no matter where you dine. Read food labels, gather nutrition brochures from your favourite dining spots and go online to restaurant and food manufacturers' websites to investigate. Also check out Good Housekeeping Calorie Counter for basic foods such as cereals, cheese and fruits, as well as popular brands.

4 Start moving

Multiple studies show that weight-loss efforts are vastly more successful when dieters reduce calories and increase their physical activity. The secret is to find activities you enjoy so that you'll want to keep doing them. And don't forget that everyday activities like gardening and walking up the stairs burn calories too. See Fitness First (Chapter 5) for lots of ideas on how to get more movement into your daily routine.

5 Change for good

Drop a Dress Size is designed to reveal your personal diet traps so that you can change your habits and (finally) shake off those extra pounds; however, if you don't modify your habits for good, you won't be able to solve your weight problems in the long term. As soon as your old eating habits return, so will the weight.

Think about adopting the strategies you learn here permanently. It will help you to maintain your ultimate goal, whether it's weight loss or healthier living.

Once you reach your desired weight, add about 100 calories to your daily intake. After a week, weigh yourself at your usual time, on your usual scales. If you have lost any weight, add another 100 calories to your daily total. Repeat until your weight remains stable – that's how much you need each day to stop losing weight and to sustain the weight loss you've accomplished.

So give it a try. Read on to learn how to overcome your weight-loss hurdles – whether they are junk-food cravings, bad exercise habits, skipping meals, emotional eating or a mixture of these or others. Once you do, you'll find that you will Drop a Dress Size in no time!

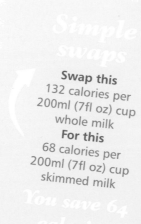

Simple swaps

Swap this
132 calories per 200ml (7fl oz) cup whole milk

For this
68 calories per 200ml (7fl oz) cup skimmed milk

You save 64 calories

The following daily calorie targets provide an easy outline for a diet. Although your exact calorie needs depend upon a variety of factors, including your height, weight and activity level, for most people, sticking to these targets will result in a steady rate of weight loss of 450g/0.5kg–1kg (1–2lb) a week.

Think of the total as your daily calorie-spending account – if you overdo it at breakfast, just have a lighter lunch. If you have an indulgent snack, cut back a bit at dinner, and so on. As long as you stay within the recommended total calories, you'll still drop pounds.

Daily calorie targets

FOR WOMEN	
BREAKFAST	350
LUNCH	500
DINNER	500
SNACK	100
OPTIONAL TREAT	100
TOTAL	1,450–1,550
FOR MEN	
BREAKFAST	450
LUNCH	600
DINNER	600
SNACK	200
OPTIONAL TREAT	200
TOTAL	1,850–2,050

Men have more lean tissue (muscle) than women, so they need more calories each day. The meals in this book fall within the calorie guidelines for women. Men will need to add about 100 calories to each meal or snack, either by eating larger portions or by rounding out meals with nutrient-dense foods. The chart on page 13 shows some easy ways to add 100 calories to any recipe or meal.

To keep your energy level up and to feel your best, fuel your body with nutrient-packed calories from foods such as fruits, vegetables, lean proteins, low-fat dairy, wholegrain breads and cereals, and judicious amounts of healthy fats such as avocado, olive oil, nuts and seeds

100-calorie options

PRODUCE	GRAINS	PROTEIN
1 medium potato	1 thick slice wholemeal bread	200ml (7fl oz) semi-skimmed milk or 25g (1oz) cheese
2 handfuls, 160g (5½oz), grapes	1 small bowl, 25g (1oz), wholegrain cereal	1 tbsp peanut butter or 2 tbsp nuts
2 apples	3 tbsp cooked wholegrain rice	3 tbsp, 100g (3½oz), cooked beans
1 banana	3 tbsp cooked wholegrain pasta	Small, 75g (3oz), skinless chicken breast
Half a small avocado	Small portion noodles 25g (1oz) uncooked weight	Small fillet, 100g (3½oz), white fish or 75g (3oz) tuna in water

(see Make the Most of Your Calories, page 10). Have the optional 100-calorie treat (see page 30) once a day, or save up those calories for a larger treat every other day, or enjoy 350-calorie treats twice a week. If you want to cut calories a little more, skip the optional treat altogether.

There's no need to cut out all fats – studies have shown that people following a low-fat diet are no more successful than those on other diets. If anything, those who include more fat – in the healthy form of nuts, olive oil or oily fish – lose more weight. This is because fat helps to keep you feeling 'full' for longer, so you are not tempted to snack between meals. So don't avoid fat, but focus on eating the right kinds of fat: unsaturated fats found in plant and nut oils such as olive, groundnut and rapeseed; nuts such as almonds, walnuts, brazils, cashews and pistachios; avocados and oily fish.

Eating in

If you want to have a healthier diet, enjoy delicious and satisfying meals, and win the war against unwanted weight, eating at home is a key strategy. It gives you the most control over your diet, and you will avoid the tempting bread baskets, fat-laden dishes and calorie-dense desserts that you find in restaurants. Restaurant servings keep getting bigger, and so do dress sizes!

Food is one of life's great pleasures – especially sharing it with family and friends – and eating at home provides you with full command over food choices and portions. You can also experiment with ingredients and try good-for-your-waistline recipes and foods. With an abundance of tips and advice, this chapter shows you how to practise good eating habits at home.

Dining well at home doesn't require you to follow a strict set of rules or give up your favourite foods. Instead, it's about making healthy, common-sense choices.

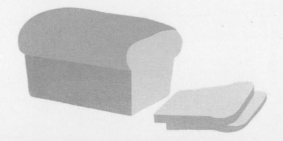

1 Detox your kitchen

Clear your cupboards, fridge and freezer of the foods you know will get you into trouble, and instead stock up on healthy and tasty options you and your family will enjoy. Conduct your own in-house taste tests – ask your family to get involved, try new, lower-calorie recipes and new foods, and gain a new (and healthy!) weight-loss perspective.

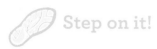

Step on it!

Omelette makeover
A few subtle changes to the ingredients of a cheese omelette can cut 202 calories and 17g (½oz) fat – but none of the taste. Instead of using 2 whole eggs and 60g (2¼oz) cheese, make an omelette with 2 whole eggs and 1 egg white plus 25g (1oz) of cheese. You won't be able to tell the difference.

2 Recipe makeovers

Substitute ingredients used in everyday cooking with healthier options and you'll slash calories – and propel yourself to success. The cooking tricks below will not only help you maintain your desired weight once you get there, but are useful things for all the family to learn.

Here are some tips for trimming excess fat and calories from home-cooked meals:

- Choose lean cuts of meat and trim all visible fat before cooking. Remove the skin from poultry before or after cooking.
- Cut back on the fat in proper gravy – just pour most of the fat out of the used roasting tin before you make gravy. Alternatively, invest in a gravy separator, which will split the fat from the meat juices so that you can pour a sin-free version over your Sunday roast.
- If a roast chicken tops your Sunday wish-list, rather than slathering it with butter before cooking, squeeze some lemon juice over the bird and drizzle with 1 tbsp olive oil. And when the chicken's cooked, remember to get rid of the skin before eating, as it is very fatty.
- A classic fore-rib of beef is high in fat – an artery-clogging 20g (¾oz) fat per 100g (3½oz). So opt for a leaner topside joint. Before roasting, sit the meat on a rack to allow much of the fat to drip into the tin during cooking, rather than leaving the meat swimming in it.
- Make skinny chips by slicing 2 large potatoes into wedges, then put them on a non-stick baking tray. Pour ½ tbsp olive oil over them, season and cook at 200°C (180°C fan oven) mark 6 for 30 minutes.
- Substitute protein-packed canned pulses, such as beans and lentils, for meat in casseroles; the dish will have fewer calories and more filling fibre.
- Use skimmed milk in a cheese sauce rather than whole milk, and replace ordinary Cheddar cheese with fuller-flavoured mature or vintage Cheddar – this will allow you to cut the amount of cheese you use by half.
- Be sparing with fat. Use non-stick pans or a non-stick cooking spray with regular pans.
- Experiment with fat-free flavourings: squeeze orange or lemon juice into stews or over meats; add citrus zest, soy sauce, fresh ginger, chilli peppers, herbs or tomato purée to your favourite recipes.
- Before roasting fish or chicken, spritz with olive oil spray before seasoning and adding herbs or spices, to minimize fat and maximize

the taste of the flavourings. Spray oil on vegetables (rather than brushing it on) to cut down on fat.

- Turn potato salad into a healthy energy booster by replacing ordinary mayonnaise with 2 tbsp reduced-calorie mayonnaise mixed with an equal amount of low-fat yogurt.
- For a healthier version of spag bol, swap regular minced beef, at 15g (½oz) fat per 100g (3½oz), for extra-lean mince, at 10g (¼oz) fat per 100g (3½oz), or turkey mince, at 7g (¼oz) fat per 100g (3½oz), then brown in a little oil. Add flavour with fresh herbs and boost the nutritional value with celery, mushrooms and carrots.
- Swap double cream in sauces for low-fat yogurt to dramatically lower the fat content of a dish. Take care not to let the sauce boil, though, as this might cause it to split.

3 Downsize your dishes

Use smaller plates and glasses for everyday meals. According to a Cornell University study, people tend to serve themselves 30 per cent more food when given large bowls and spoons. And research at the Food and Brand Lab at the University of Illinois found that people who used short, wide glasses poured 76 per cent more soda, milk or juice than when they used tall, slender ones.

No need to buy new, though: simply swap your dinner plate for a side plate or salad plate, or a large glass for a small glass. Or, if you have fashionably oversized dishes and glasses, use a measuring jug or measuring cups to familiarize yourself with calorie-controlled portions and keep these studies in mind as you ladle out the servings.

Emotion-related eating

Overeating can be a way of coping with stress, but you can conquer it. Work out what triggers your eating: do you munch when you are sad, lonely, angry, bored or guilt-ridden? Whatever your triggers, an important part of breaking the habit is finding out what's pushing you to turn to food. Eliminate stressors where possible and start using other means to cope. When you recognize an urge to eat, ask yourself if you are truly hungry. Physical hunger tends to be gradual, whereas an appetite caused by emotional reasons usually comes on suddenly.

4 Control cravings

Whether it's chocolate or chips, ice cream or whipped cream, the foods people crave have one thing in common – they are calorie-dense, a Tufts University study recently confirmed. But, in that study, the researchers also noted that while virtually everyone had cravings, the dieters in the group who successfully lost weight or kept it off gave in to their must-haves – but just less often.

5 Pay attention

A recent study showed that Americans (and the British are much the same) use external cues, such as waiting until their television programme is over, to stop eating, unlike the don't-get-fat French, who rely on internal messages, such as feeling full. We're also susceptible to social influences. Many of us keep eating until almost everyone at the table is finished. If you tend to finish before your family, keep the salad bowl in front of you to pick from, rather than having extra pasta and sauce.

KITCHEN CLEAN-UP

Here's a list of items to purge from your kitchen – and, following that, our favourite must-haves to stock up on. Donate unopened foods to a local charity, or use up what you have to hand and then replace with our picks.

Items to purge

Throw away high-calorie, nutrient-poor foods including:

- Crisps
- Salted nuts
- Chocolates and sweets
- Snacks (like breadsticks and crackers)
- Biscuits
- Sugary cereals
- Pastries
- Cakes
- White bread
- Dips
- Creamy salad dressing and sauces
- Mayonnaise
- Cream
- Sausages and burgers
- Bacon, pancetta and lardons
- Cured meats such as salami and chorizo
- Canned meats
- Squash, fizzy drinks and juice drinks

Must-haves for your fridge

Add these fridge essentials to your weekly shopping list so that they are always to hand:

- Seasonal fresh fruit and vegetables (page 82)
- Cheese – lower-fat cheeses such as Edam, feta and Gouda, or small amounts of full-fat strong cheeses such as mature Cheddar or Parmesan to provide a flavour lift (see page 86)
- Hummus
- Semi-skimmed or skimmed milk (or soya milk) and yogurt (page 86)
- Eggs (for more on cholesterol and eggs, see page 87)
- Fresh chicken, turkey and lean meat (see page 81)

 Step on it!

Look for unsweetened choices
It's easy to pick up a jar of pasta sauce, a carton of soup or a packet of breakfast cereal without realizing that a lot of sugar has been added. One leading fresh soup, for example, has 6 tsp of sugar in a 600ml carton, while a pasta sauce from another manufacturer has 6½ tsp in a 500g jar. For foods like these, which often taste great without being sweetened, be sure to check the ingredients list and look for unsweetened or only slightly sweetened alternatives.

Must-haves for your food cupboard

Once you've cleaned out the shelves, it's time to fill them with healthy options:

- Whole grains such as wholewheat pasta, wholegrain rice and noodles
- Low-fat sauces such as pasta sauce, salsa, soy sauce, etc.
- Wholemeal bread, wraps, rolls, pitta breads, tortillas, etc.
- Canned beans, salmon and tuna (in water, not oil), tomatoes, low-fat soups and fruit in juice
- Nuts, seeds and occasional treats (pages 30–31)

Must-have condiments

Add low-calorie flavour with these extras:

- Mustard (wholegrain, Dijon, etc.)
- Spray salad dressings
- Vinegar (balsamic, sherry, red wine, white wine, etc.)
- Oils (good options include olive, rapeseed, safflower and flaxseed oils)
- Herbs and spices, fresh and dried

Must-haves for your freezer

A quick, healthy meal or treat is always just minutes away:

- Healthy frozen ready meals
- Boneless, skinless chicken breasts and fish fillets are easy everyday dinner solutions when paired with a quick sauce
- Bags of frozen fruits (such as raspberries, mixed berries) and vegetables (such as spinach, peas)
- Portions of home-made, low-fat soups and casseroles
- Frozen yogurt

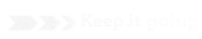

Home cooking is a healthier way of eating than using ready meals – and something we have long championed at Good Housekeeping – but sadly, some of the tastiest dishes are laden with fat. Here's how small tweaks to your family's favourite meals can give big results:

Chicken Korma

This curry tastes just as good if you swap the double cream for quark (a low-fat, soft, creamy cheese) and cut the amount of coconut cream – it contains 20g (¾oz) fat per 100ml (3½fl oz).

Marinate 4 chopped, skinless chicken breasts in 1 tbsp sunflower oil, a little grated ginger, 2 tsp garam masala, 1 tsp turmeric and 3 tbsp quark. Leave in the fridge for at least 20 minutes or preferably overnight. Spray a non-stick pan with oil and cook a chopped onion for 10 minutes, or until soft and golden. Add a crushed garlic clove and a finely chopped red chilli, and cook for 1 minute. Stir in the chicken and marinade. Cook, stirring, for 5 minutes or until lightly golden. Add 150ml (5fl oz) water, season, bring to the boil, then simmer, covered, for 15–20 minutes. Stir in 200g (7oz) quark, 1 tbsp coconut cream and 25g (1oz) ground almonds. Garnish with flaked almonds and fresh coriander. Serve with rice. (Serves 4, 324 calories per serving.)

Calories saved per portion = 160

Shepherd's Pie

You can really make a difference to the fat in your favourite shepherd's pie recipe by mashing the cooked potatoes with skimmed instead of whole milk and stirring in 1–2 tbsp reduced-fat soft cheese instead of butter (which adds only 4g (⅛oz) fat per tbsp rather than 25g (1oz) fat per tbsp). (Serves 4, 530 calories per serving.)

Calories saved per portion = 150

A Healthy Burger

Try making burgers with turkey mince. It's lean, tastes great and will cut the fat of a normal beefburger by more than half!

Pulse 450g (1lb) turkey mince, 2 shallots and a small handful of fresh parsley in a food processor. Stir in 3 tbsp spiced fruit chutney, 50g (2oz) dried breadcrumbs, the zest of 1 lemon, some seasoning and a beaten egg. Shape into four patties and chill for 20 minutes. Heat a non-stick frying pan over a medium heat, then spray with oil. Fry the burgers for 5 minutes each side or until cooked through. (Serves 4, 281 calories per serving.)

Calories saved per portion = 140

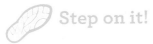
Cauliflower Cheese

Put 4 tbsp flour into a pan with 600ml (1 pint)
skimmed milk, a little grated nutmeg and ¼ tsp
cayenne pepper. Bring to the boil, whisking,
until thickened. Simmer for 3 minutes, then stir
in ½ tsp each wholegrain and English mustard
and 100g (3½oz) grated half-fat mature
Cheddar cheese. Pour over cooked cauliflower.
Mix 50g (2oz) cheese with 2 tbsp dried
breadcrumbs; sprinkle over the cauliflower
mixture. Grill for 3–4 minutes until golden.
(Serves 4, 285 calories per serving.)

Calories saved per portion = 200

Lemon Tart

This delicious dessert makes a glorious tea-time
treat or a sumptuous end to a dinner party.

For the pastry, whizz together 150g (5oz) flour
and 60g (2¼oz) butter until it resembles fine

breadcrumbs. (Alternatively, rub the butter into
the flour in a large bowl by hand or using a
pastry cutter, to resemble fine crumbs.) Add
1 tbsp oil, 2 tbsp icing sugar, 1 large egg yolk
and 1 tbsp water and whizz again, or stir with a
fork, until combined. Roll out on a lightly
floured surface to make a circle large enough to
fit a 20.5cm (8in) flan ring. Line with
greaseproof paper and fill with baking beans.
Bake at 200°C (180°C fan oven) mark 6 for 15
minutes. Remove from the oven and remove the
beans and greaseproof paper, then return to
the oven for 5 minutes. For the filling, mix
together 1 egg, 4 egg yolks, 150g (5oz) sugar,
150ml (¼ pint) half-fat crème fraîche, and the
grated zest and juice of 3 lemons. Reduce the
temperature to 150°C (130°C fan oven) mark 2
and pour the lemon mixture into the tart case.
Bake for 1 hour, or until the filling is just set and
the pastry is golden brown. (Serves 4, 299
calories per serving – cuts into 8 slices.)

Calories saved per portion = 100

Chocolate Brownies

Here's how to make indulgent but low-fat
brownies for an occasional treat:

Whisk 4 eggs, 50ml (2fl oz) sunflower oil, 150g
(5oz) light muscovado sugar and 1 tsp vanilla
extract. Fold in 250g (9oz) melted dark
chocolate, 75g (3oz) plain flour, ¼ tsp baking
powder and 1 tbsp cocoa powder. Pour into a
lined 20cm (8in) square tin and bake at 200°C
(180°C fan oven) mark 6 for 20 minutes. (Makes
20, 180 calories each.)

Calories saved per portion = 150

DECODING BREAKFAST

It's no secret that breakfast is the most important meal of the day. In fact, research shows that breakfast-eaters typically consume about 100 fewer calories during the course of the day – that's a 4.5kg (10lb) over a year – and weigh less than those who forgo food in the morning. Here's how to make it fit into your schedule – and how eating the right breakfast can help you to Drop a Dress Size.

These healthy ways to start your day are ready in under 10 minutes and add up to roughly 350 calories each.

Make-at-Home Muesli

Mix together 40g (1½oz) oats, 1 tbsp sultanas, 1 tbsp flaked almonds and 1 tbsp sunflower or pumpkin seeds. Serve with skimmed milk, a dollop of low-fat yogurt and some fresh sliced strawberries. (Serves 1.)

> Eating a healthy breakfast boosts your memory and mood, helps you concentrate, reduces your cholesterol levels and cuts your chances of developing diabetes or having a heart attack.

Banana Cinnamon Porridge

Mix 50g (2oz) oats, ½ tsp ground cinnamon and 350ml (12fl oz) skimmed milk in a pan. Bring to the boil and simmer for about 5 minutes, stirring frequently. Serve topped with a sliced banana and a drizzle of honey. (Serves 1.)

Yogurt with Dried Fruit Compote

The day before, combine the zest and freshly squeezed juice of 1 orange with 2 tbsp honey and 300ml (½ pint) water in a pan. Bring the mixture to the boil, then add 250g (9oz) of dried fruit (such as ready-to-eat figs, apricots and prunes) and simmer, covered, for 5–10 minutes until they become plump and soft. Allow

Simple swaps

Swap this
232 calories per bagel
For this
77 calories per crumpet

You save 155 calories

 ## Step on it!

Add fruit to your cereal
Adding fresh sliced berries, bananas, peaches or whatever is in season to your bowl of wholegrain cereal is a wonderful way to sneak more fruit into your diet. It not only adds a sweet flavour but it also provides lots of satisfying fibre.

to cool and keep covered in the fridge until you are ready to serve. (Serves 4.) The next day, stir a portion of fruit compote into 150ml (¼ pint) fat free Greek yogurt to make one serving.

Fruit Smoothie

In a smoothie-maker, blender or food processor, whizz together a small cupful of crushed ice, a 125ml pot of raspberry yogurt, 150ml (¼ pint) cranberry juice drink, 50g (2oz) raspberries and a little orange juice. (Serves 1.)

Scrambled Eggs on Wholemeal Toast

Using a fork, whisk 2 eggs in a microwave-proof bowl with a little milk, seasoning and 1 tsp oil. Put in the microwave and cook on full power for 1 minute. Remove and whisk lightly with a fork. Return to the microwave and cook for a further 30 seconds. Stir. The eggs should be lightly set. Leave to stand for 1 minute. Meanwhile, toast a thin slice of wholemeal bread. Put on a plate and pile the eggs on top.

Need to eat on the move? Make these tasty bars the day before – they'll fuel you through the morning.

Breakfast Bars

Put 175g (6oz) oats in a bowl and combine with 75g (3oz) plain flour, 150g (5oz) dried fruit mixture (such as raisins, dates, apricots, figs, apple and pineapple) and 3 heaped tbsp honey, warmed in a pan until runny, 1 egg and 175ml (6fl oz) apple juice. Press the mixture into a lightly oiled 18 × 28cm (7 × 11in) baking tin. Bake at 180°C (160°C fan oven) mark 4 for 20–25 minutes until golden. Cut into bars while still warm. (Makes 12.)

Still want that fry-up? Here's how:

Swap a fried pork sausage (139 calories) for a grilled Quorn sausage (69 calories)
Saves 70 calories

Swap a grilled streaky bacon rasher (67 calories) for a back bacon rasher (43 calories)
Saves 24 calories

Swap a fried egg (107 calories) for a poached egg (74 calories)
Saves 33 calories

Swap fried bread (274 calories) for wholemeal toast with a scraping of butter (116 calories)
Saves 158 calories

Total saving = 285 calories

What do you do when you find yourself at home at lunchtime? Do you make a quick sandwich? Or eat yesterday's leftovers? Or perhaps you skip lunch completely and end up snacking all afternoon. Here are some midday ideas for when you're at home and trying to keep a your calories in check.

The 450-calorie sandwich

A sandwich doesn't have to be loaded with fat and calories, especially when it's made at home. Here's how to construct the perfect sandwich:

Bread, 200 calories: Choose wholegrain or wholemeal bread for your sandwich – but watch the size. A big sub roll, for example, might contain up to 500 calories! Instead, choose two slices of wholemeal sandwich bread or one small roll equal to about 200 calories.

Butter/substitutes, 50 calories: A thin scraping of butter (around 1 teaspoon/5g per slice) stops a filling making the bread soggy. Want a healthier option? Swap butter for an olive oil spread for its heart-healthy monounsaturated fats. Alternatively, spread your bread with naturally low-fat mustard. For a creamier spread, mix low-fat yogurt with a little mustard.

Cheese, 50 calories: You can add cheese to your sandwich without breaking the calorie bank: 20g (¾oz) of feta, for example, is only 50 calories; 1 tbsp Philadelphia Light cream cheese has 47 calories. Other lower-fat options include mozzarella at 52 calories per 20g (¾oz) and Brie at 68 calories per 20g (¾oz). Look for any variety of reduced-fat cheese with about 250–300 calories per 100g (3½oz).

Meat/fish, 100 calories: Cured meats, such as ham and bacon, are high in calories and salt. Cured meat or sausage sandwiches should be occasional indulgences, not everyday fare. Look for lower-calorie alternatives such as lean beef, chicken breast, turkey breast and tuna. Aim for about 100 calories of lean protein, which is about five slices of meat (each deli slice is about 20 calories) or a 75g (3oz) serving of tuna in water.

Dressings, 50 calories: Instead of high-fat mayonnaise, use a reduced-fat variety and add some chopped fresh herbs for flavour. Chutney or relish, delicious by itself or when blended with light mayonnaise or mustard, adds a delectable sweet-and-spicy dimension to a sandwich.

Vegetables, no limit: Go wild – add spinach, lettuce, red pepper, onions, cucumber, mushrooms, tomato or any other fresh vegetable for extra flavour, fibre and virtually no calories. Avoid vegetables packed or roasted in oil, which pack unwanted calories.

Total calorie goal: about 450

Now, to finish your meal, add a piece of fruit (a banana, pear or nectarine, for example). Voilà – the perfect lunch to help you Drop a Dress Size!

Did you know?

The average person eats 230 sandwiches a year. That's a lot of bread and probably BLT too – make sure you stick to healthy options.

The low-down on sandwich spreads and dressings

Spread/dressing	Grams of fat	Calories per tbsp
Butter (10g)	8	74
Polyunsaturated margarine (10g)	8	75
Olive oil spread (10g)	6	54
Reduced fat spread (10g)	4	35
Mayonnaise 25g (1oz)	23	207
Pesto 25g (1oz)	11	138
Mango chutney 25g (1oz)	0	57
Light mayonnaise 25g (1oz)	9	88
French dressing 15g (½oz)	11	98
Branston pickle 25g (1oz)	0	33
Barbecue sauce 20g (¾oz)	0	19
Hummus 25g (1oz)	7	80
Ketchup 20g (¾oz)	0	23
Mustard 10g (¼oz)	1	11
Salsa 40g (1½oz)	0	13

At about 500 calories each, the tempting dinners in this section will help you to lose weight and keep you satisfied too.

Crusted Cod with Grilled Tomatoes

Preheat the grill. Heat 1 tsp oil in a small frying pan that can be used under the grill. Fry a 150g (5oz) boneless fillet of cod, skin-side down in the pan for 3 minutes. Meanwhile, whizz a standard slice of stale white bread, about 25g (1oz), in a food processor until it forms breadcrumbs (or coarsely grate it instead). Put the breadcrumbs into a bowl with 1 tbsp freshly chopped parsley (or 1 tsp dried mixed herbs), the finely grated zest of ¼ lemon and 1 tsp olive oil. Carefully lift the part-cooked fish on to a baking sheet and top with the herby mixture. Next to the cod, put a 75g (3oz) bunch of cherry tomatoes on the vine. Grill for 5 minutes until the fish is cooked and the tomatoes have just burst. Serve immediately with 175g (6oz) boiled new potatoes and salad. (Serves 1, 460 calories.)

WRAP IT UP

Cooking 'en papillote' might have a fancy French name but it just means cooking in a parcel and is a great technique for making single servings. Simply put a portion of meat (chicken is ideal) or fish on a large square of foil or baking parchment, add some thinly sliced vegetables and aromatics (garlic/ginger/chilli/fresh herbs), fold up the edges of the foil or baking parchment and pour in a little water or stock. Seal, then cook in the oven at 180°C (160°C fan oven) mark 4, or steam in a steamer, for 15 minutes for fish or 30 minutes for chicken (depending on size) until ready.

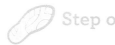 Step on it!

Sample more seafood

Follow a low-cal diet that includes more fish than meat and the chances are that you'll drop more pounds than you would otherwise – at least, that's according to a study published in the *International Journal of Obesity*. One possible explanation is that, gram for gram, fish has fewer calories than almost all cuts of beef, pork and skin-on poultry. Researchers theorize that omega-3 fatty acids, the polyunsaturated fats abundant in cold-water fish such as salmon and mackerel, switch on the fat-burning process in cells – provided that you also exercise.

Gruyère and Watercress Omelette

Heat ½ tbsp vegetable oil over a low heat in a small frying pan. Lightly beat 2–3 large eggs (depending on hunger!), season and add to the pan. Use a spatula to move the eggs around for the first 30 seconds. Next, top the egg with a small handful of roughly chopped watercress and 25g (1oz) grated Gruyère cheese. Continue cooking until the base of the omelette is golden (check with the spatula) and the cheese is melting. Fold in half and serve with a medium baked potato, 175g (6oz), with 10g butter and a green salad. (Serves 1, 485 calories.)

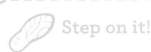 Step on it!

Fancy a chip?
Make your own chips from fresh potatoes – frozen chips cool down in the hot oil during cooking, so they don't seal so quickly and will therefore absorb more fat. Per 100g (3½oz) cooked portion, frozen fried chips have 273 calories and 13.5g (½oz) fat, whereas home-made ones have only 189 calories and 5g (¼oz) fat.

Spiced Yogurt Chicken

In a large bowl, stir together 200g (7oz) fat-free Greek yogurt, 2 crushed garlic cloves, 1cm (½in) piece peeled and grated fresh root ginger, 1 tsp garam masala, ½ tsp each ground cinnamon and chilli powder, ¼ tsp ground turmeric, 1 tbsp vegetable oil, 1½ tsp lemon juice and some seasoning. Add 8 skinless and boneless chicken thigh fillets, 75g (3oz) each, and stir to coat. Cover and chill for 1 hour, if you have time. Preheat the oven to 200°C (180°C fan oven) mark 6. Tip the chicken and marinade into a roasting tin and cook for 20 minutes until the chicken is cooked. Meanwhile, in a small bowl stir together 100g (3½oz) fat-free Greek yogurt and 2 tbsp mango chutney. Serve the chicken with the mango yogurt and some plain boiled wholegrain rice. (Serves 4, 454 calories per serving.)

Risotto Verde

Heat 1 tbsp oil in a large pan over a medium heat. Fry 1 finely chopped onion for 10 minutes, then stir in 300g (11oz) risotto rice and cook for 1 minute, followed by 75ml (2½fl oz) white wine (optional). Starting with 1 litre (1¾ pints) hot vegetable stock, add a ladleful of stock to the rice pan and stir until the stock is absorbed. Continue adding the stock and stirring until the rice is tender – about 15–20 minutes. Add 150g (5oz) frozen soya beans and 1 chopped courgette 10 minutes before the risotto is due to be ready and 150g (5oz) frozen peas for the final 5 minutes of cooking. When the risotto is ready, stir in 3 tbsp mixed freshly chopped parsley, chives and mint. Serve topped with a little grated Parmesan (optional). (Serves 4, 412 calories per serving.)

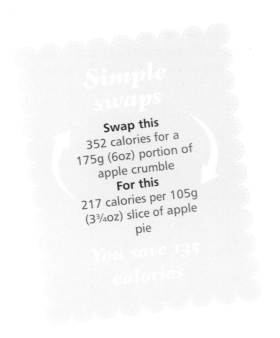

Simple swaps

Swap this
352 calories for a 175g (6oz) portion of apple crumble
For this
217 calories per 105g (3¾oz) slice of apple pie

You save 135 calories

NO MORE TEARS

Buy a few extra onions next time you go to the shops. Peel and finely chop as normal, then freeze in a freezer bag (lay as flat as possible). Next time a recipe calls for part of a chopped onion, simply use some from your frozen stash.

One-pan Creamy Spring Chicken Supper

Fry 1 skinless chicken breast in 1 tsp olive oil for 5 minutes on each side until golden. Add a little garlic, then stir in 100g (3½oz) new potatoes and 75ml (2½fl oz) stock. Cover and simmer for another 10 minutes. Add 50g (2oz) each of peas and broccoli, cover and cook for 5 minutes. Check whether the chicken is cooked before stirring in a little Dijon mustard and 1 tbsp yogurt and crumbling 20g (¾oz) goat's cheese over the top. (Serves 1, 422 calories.)

Chicken Traybake

Preheat the oven to 200°C (180°C fan oven) mark 6. Heat 1 tbsp oil in a large roasting tin, then fry 4 × 125g (4oz) skinless chicken breasts for 5 minutes until golden. Take off the heat and stir in 2 chopped sweet potatoes and 2 deseeded and chopped peppers. Season well. Roast for 20 minutes, then add 4 quartered tomatoes, 1 tbsp fresh (or ½ tbsp dried) oregano and 75g (3oz) each roughly chopped pitted black olives and sun-dried tomatoes. Return to oven for 10 minutes or until the tomatoes are softening. Serve with a crisp green salad. (Serves 4, 426 calories per serving.)

Light Lamb Stew

Heat ½ tbsp vegetable oil over a high heat in a large pan. Brown 400g (14oz) lamb neck fillet cut into 2cm (¾in) dice (do this in batches if necessary). Add 4 halved shallots, 1 sliced leek and 1 chopped carrot and fry for 3–5 minutes. Stir in 50g (2oz) pearl barley and 750ml (1¼ pints) lamb or chicken stock. Simmer gently, covered, for 20 minutes or until the lamb is tender, adding ½ pointed cabbage, shredded, 5 minutes before the end of the cooking time. Stir in 100g (3½oz) frozen peas and a small handful of fresh mint. Heat through and check the seasoning. Serve with 4 small boiled new potatoes per person and salad. (Serves 4, 450 calories per serving.)

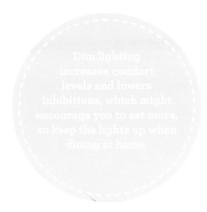

Dim lighting increases comfort levels and lowers inhibitions, which might encourage you to eat more, so keep the lights up when dining at home.

Creamy Chicken Pasta

Cook 350g (12oz) dried tagliatelle according to the pack instructions. Meanwhile, heat ½ tbsp oil in a large frying pan and fry 350g (12oz) chicken strips for 3–4 minutes until a light golden colour (do this in batches if necessary). Pour in 175ml (6fl oz) strong chicken stock, bring to a simmer and cook for 5 minutes until the chicken is cooked through. Stir in 5 tbsp half-fat crème fraîche, 1 tbsp dried sage and 1 deseeded and finely chopped red chilli. Drain the pasta and add to the chicken sauce, then stir in 50g (2oz) roughly chopped rocket. Check the seasoning and serve topped with a little grated Parmesan, if you like. (Serves 4, 448 calories per serving.)

Simple swaps

Swap this
343 calories for 1 slice, 65g (2½oz), Victoria sponge
For this
229 calories per toasted tea cake with 5g (⅛oz) butter
You save 114 calories

Think you need to give up snacking to lose weight? On the contrary, the Drop a Dress Size plan has two 100-calorie snacks/optional treats built in. Here are our favourites, both savoury and sweet, which will help you stay on track. (You'll also find more snacks in the weekday planners.)

50-calorie munchies

Savoury snacks These tasty snack ideas will help keep hunger at bay, and at about 50 calories each, you can have two to four per day:

- 1 rice cake with 1 tbsp mashed avocado
- 1½ tbsp low-fat hummus with ½ small red pepper, sliced for dipping
- 5 almonds
- 10 carrot sticks with 2 tbsp salsa for dipping
- 1 handful, 10g (¼oz), Tyrell's lightly salted popcorn

Sweet snacks Satisfy your sugar cravings with these quick, low-cal fixes:

 Step on it!

Smarter snacks
Your twice-daily 100-calorie Drop a Dress Size snacks can be indulgent treats (biscuits, crisps) or a healthy way to stave off hunger (fruit, vegetables, yogurt, nuts, wholegrain snacks) until your next meal. If your favourite treat does not come in 100-calorie pre-packaged servings, divide it into 100-calorie portions yourself.

Mix 250ml (9fl oz) brewed coffee with 250ml (9fl oz) heated skimmed milk, and pour into a cup. Add a sprinkle of cinnamon or cocoa powder for a sweet flavour, if you like.

Or you can whip up a low-fat latte instead – even if you don't have an espresso machine at home. Combine 25–50g (1–2oz) powdered espresso, to taste, with 250ml (9fl oz) skimmed milk, then heat in the microwave for 1 minute. Serve.

- 1 Hartley's jelly pot (no added sugar; any flavour)
- 1 meringue nest
- 1 packet sugar-free Polo mints
- 2 dates
- 1 low-calorie hot chocolate drink

23 M&Ms	= 1 handful, 35g (1¼oz), raisins
	= a 125g pot low-fat fruit yogurt
	= 1 large punnet, 350g (12oz), strawberries

The 100-calorie comparison

Low-density foods have relatively few calories compared to their weight. These foods are high in water or fibre and add bulk to meals, allowing you to feel satisfied with fewer calories; for example, all the foods below can be diet-friendly snacks, but the strawberries will leave you feeling the fullest.

100-calorie munches

Each of these tasty nibbles has about 100 calories, so you can have one or two a day:

Sweet treats
- 25 Jelly Belly jelly beans
- 1 McVitie's chocolate digestive
- 1 Kellogg's Special K red berry bar
- 1 Müller Light strawberry yogurt
- 1 Alpen Light chocolate and orange bar
- 2 squares, 20g (¾oz), milk chocolate
- 2 Jaffa cakes
- 1 Skinny Cow mint double choc stick

Swap this
364 calories for a Starbucks grande mocha
For this
90 calories for a home-made café au lait

Step on it!

Stock your house with calorie-controlled snacks
You don't have to eliminate your favourite not-so-healthy snacks. Supermarket shelves are chock-full of 100-calorie packs of biscuits, crisps, crackers, cereal bars and more. Although they cost more than a larger pack of the same product, they make it easier for you to indulge without overeating.

You can also think of them as training wheels for dieting: 100-calorie snack packs can help you learn how to keep indulgences in check. In a study by the University of Colorado in Denver, 59 adults ate snack foods for two weeks. Half the group munched from 100-calorie packs for one week, followed by the same treats from larger packs for the next; for the other half, the order was reversed.

Outcome: the volunteers who were first 'trained' with small packs took 852 fewer calories from the big packs. You can learn to recognize the right amount, say the study's authors, who suggest buying the 100-calorie bags of snacks (or measuring out that amount of a favourite). Then, whenever you encounter that snack food, you'll know what a 'safe' portion is.

You can get fit without setting foot in a gym. These easy moves are designed to tone your body and can be done on a mat in the comfort of your own home.

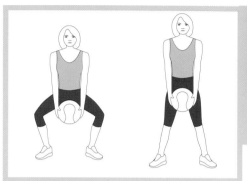

Plié squats

Stand with your feet a little wider than shoulder-width apart, and with toes and knees pointing out at a 45° angle. Hold a medicine ball (or a medium-sized ball) and squat down until your thighs are parallel to the floor. Keep your back straight and head looking forwards. Return to the starting position. Repeat 12–15 times.

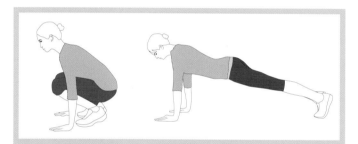

Squat thrusts

From a standing position, crouch down to a squat position with your hands on the ground shoulder-width apart, near your feet. From this position, jump back with your feet so you're in a press-up position. Then jump forwards, back to your squat position, with your hands still on the floor. Repeat 10 times.

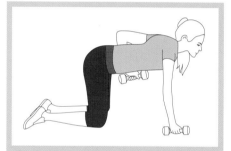

Kneeling row

Kneeling on all fours, hold a weight in your left hand and support your body weight on your right hand. Pull the weight up towards your armpit. Hold for a second before lowering the weight. Keep your back still and straight. Repeat 10–12 times.

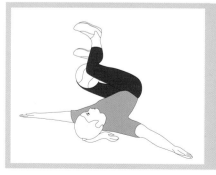

Medicine ball hip roll

Lie on your back with a medicine ball (or medium-sized ball) between your knees. Lift your feet off the floor, forming a 90° angle at your hips and knees. Roll your hips over to the left until the leg touches the floor. Use your side muscles to lift the legs back up to the starting position. Repeat, rolling to the right side. Alternate to the right and left sides 8–10 times.

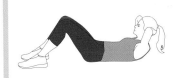
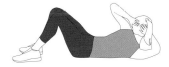
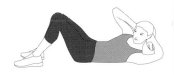

Ab crossover

Lie on your back with your hands by the side of your head and your legs raised, knees bent at a 90° angle. Bring your left elbow towards your right knee. Return to the starting position and then repeat on the other side. Alternate sides and repeat 12–15 times.

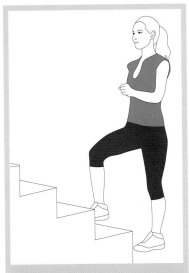

Step-ups

Stand up straight in front of a low bench or the first step of the stairs. Step up with one leg and then the other. Return to the starting position. Repeat 10–12 times with the right leg leading, then repeat 10–12 times with the left leg leading.

Seated overhead triceps extension

Sit on a stability/Swiss ball or chair and hold a weight with both hands. Extend your arms to the ceiling, keeping them close to your ears. This is the starting position. Lower the weight behind your head until it touches your shoulders. Straighten your arms back to the starting position. Repeat 12–15 times.

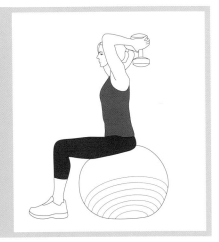

Leg lift

Lie on your right side and extend your left leg forwards to form a 45° angle, with your toes touching the floor. Lift your left leg up off the floor until it is level with your hips. Lower your leg back down to the floor. Repeat 12–15 times before changing sides.

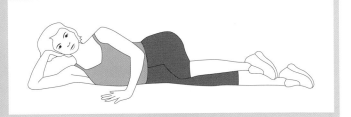

FAT-BUSTING WEEKDAY MEAL PLANNER

	MONDAY	TUESDAY	WEDNESDAY	THURSDAY	FRIDAY
BREAKFAST (about 350 calories)	Make-at-Home Muesli with skimmed milk (p. 22)	150ml (½ pint) fat-free Greek yogurt with 100g (3½oz) berries, 1 tbsp flaked almonds and 2 tsp honey	40g (1½oz) bran flakes with 150ml (¼ pint) skimmed milk and 1 banana	2 slices of wholemeal toast with 2 tsp butter and Marmite; café au lait (p. 30)	1 poached egg on 2 slices of wholemeal toast; 1 piece of fruit
LUNCH (about 500 calories)	Tuna Salad (p. 137) with a wholemeal roll and 2 tsp butter; 1 piece of fruit	Chicken and watercress sandwich with 2 tsp low-fat mayonnaise; 80g (3¼oz) fresh berries	Tomato, Pepper and Orange Soup (p. 141) with 1 wholemeal roll and 2 tsp butter; 1 x 125g pot low-fat yogurt	Smoked Mackerel Citrus Salad (p. 138) with 1 slice wholemeal bread and 1 tsp butter; 1 piece fresh fruit	Leafy salad with 1 sliced avocado, 1 hard-boiled egg and 1 tbsp low-fat mayonnaise
DINNER (about 500 calories)	Chicken Stir-fry with Noodles (p. 130); 75g (3oz) strawberries with 1 tbsp fat-free Greek yogurt	Tomato and Butter Bean Stew (p. 134) with a 175g (6oz) baked potato, 2 tsp butter and 1 tbsp grated cheese	Prawn and Vegetable Pilau (p. 134); 150g (5oz) fruit salad with 1 tbsp fat-free Greek yogurt	Chickpea Curry (p. 139) with 4 tbsp cooked wholegrain rice	Turkey and Broccoli Stir-fry (p. 141) with 4 tbsp cooked wholegrain noodles; 150g (5oz) fresh fruit
SNACK (about 100 calories)	½ mango and 1 apple	10 almonds	1 rice cake with 1 Dairylea slice	1 slice of wholemeal toast with a scrape of butter	1 Müller Light cherry yogurt

Step on it!

Add a dash of chilli sauce to your meal
In a 2010 study, scientists at the University of California found that people who consumed meals containing chilli burned up almost twice as much energy for several hours afterwards compared with the placebo group. Over a month, their bodies became more efficient at burning fat.

Eat off the last few pounds with these long-term strategies:

• Keep a food diary. Sometimes there's a difference between what you think you're eating and what you're really putting into your mouth.
• Don't be a yo-yo dieter or crash-dieter. Consistent lifestyle changes are the key to permanent weight loss.
• Check your portion sizes. Plates piled high, even with healthy foods, will pile on the pounds. A protein portion, for example, should be no bigger than the size of an iPhone (see Practise Portion Control on page 56).
• Eat slowly, chewing every mouthful and allowing yourself to start feeling full rather than bolting food down and going for second helpings.
• Don't cut out food groups, unless you have a medical reason not to eat them. Aim for a mix of everything – just keep fats, sugar and refined carbohydrates to a minimum.

Getting down to work

When you start your workday, you may have the best of intentions. You resolve to eat a healthy breakfast at home but you're late so you grab a croissant on the way to work instead. Perhaps you plan to go for a brisk walk at lunchtime – but then a client calls unexpectedly and you're stuck on the phone during your lunch hour. Later, you'd like to turn down a slice of your colleague's birthday cake, but wouldn't it be rude to refuse?

Relax. An occasional slip-up isn't the end of the world – not if you're sticking to the Drop a Dress Size plan. Incorporate the simple strategies on the following pages into your working life and you'll be on your way to a slimmer you.

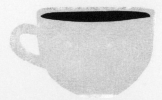

1 Partner up

Ask your colleagues – there are probably a few of them who also want to Drop a Dress Size – to form a weight-loss team. Ask team members to bring healthy lunch dishes to share on certain days, take walks during coffee breaks or at lunchtime, and exchange low-calorie recipes. Create an e-mail group to track the team's weekly loss of pounds, the number of minutes exercised and your favourite weight-loss tips.

2 Pack it

Instead of eating lunch out, where you're more likely to give in to calorie-filled choices, bring your lunch to work whenever possible. Don't think you have time? Try packing something for yourself while you're making your kids' lunches. For grab-and-go lunches the whole week through, keep your freezer stocked with figure-friendly frozen options or measure dinner leftovers into single-serving packs to take to work. If you like to socialize with your colleagues at lunchtime, encourage them to bring a packed lunch too. The bonus? You'll save money and time by eating in – and you can use the rest of your lunch hour to take a quick, energizing walk before getting back to work.

There will be days, of course, when packing a lunch isn't an option: you'll be going out for a colleague's birthday or you'll have a lunchtime work meeting. This doesn't mean that you have to throw your diet out of the window. As often as possible, choose foods that are nutrient-dense for energy (like sandwiches with wholemeal bread and lean meat), fibre-packed to curb hunger (like salads, vegetables and fruits), and calorie-controlled for weight loss. You'll thereby offset any less stellar choices you make and set yourself up for long-term Drop a Dress Size success.

Vending machine know-how

If you know that occasionally you'll fall victim to the lure of the vending machine (almost no one's immune), make your decisions ahead of time so your choices are waistline-friendly. Scan the offerings and then do some investigating – look up calories and ingredients online or read the nutrition facts labels in the supermarket, then select items with the lowest number of calories and the most nutrition. And remember, the more filling fibre a food contains, the better. Nuts, wholegrain cereal or granola bars (based on oats), trail mix, dried fruit or low-fat milkshakes are all good picks.

3 Mix it up

Perhaps you're in a rut – on your way to work, you always stop at the local coffee shop for a mocha and a pastry, or when 3.00 p.m. comes around, you take a trip to the vending machine for a bag of crisps. Recognize your routines and replace them with healthier habits: for example, swap a mocha for a low-cal skinny latte, and instead of crisps, munch on low-fat microwaved popcorn. Even small changes to your rituals can make big changes to your waistline.

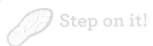
4 Build a snack arsenal

Snacking not only keeps energy levels up but it also staves off hunger until the next meal. But sometimes it's easy to get caught up in a day's duties and deadlines without refuelling. Keep low-cal snacks in your bag, desk drawer, locker or workplace fridge so that you're less likely to sabotage your Drop a Dress Size efforts when you get a snack attack at work.

5 Work it out

Australian researchers examined data on nearly 1,600 male and female full-time office workers. They found that workers sat for an average of more than three hours a day, with 25 per cent of them sedentary for more than six hours a day. A high total in daily sitting time was associated with a 68 per cent increased risk of being overweight or obese. Get physical to compensate for your sedentary workday. Join a gym, take an early morning run, find time for fitness fun with your family and use the tips and tricks in this book to incorporate more movement into your life.

Swap this
135 calories per 330ml can cola
For this
3 calories per 300ml can diet cola

Getting the kids ready for school, walking the dog, making yourself presentable for a day at work – there are so many excuses to skip a healthy breakfast in favour of a muffin and a latte from a coffee shop. Our breakfast choices remove the obstacles: these are quick and easy meals to enjoy at home, pack up and eat on the run, or nibble at your desk when you arrive at the office.

To guarantee that you never bypass this meal again, here are 12 healthy ways to start your day. Each of these morning options adds up to roughly 350 calories.

Easy at-home breakfasts

Berry yogurt Combine one 125g pot natural low-fat yogurt with a big handful of berries (such as strawberries or blueberries). Drizzle with 1 tbsp honey and top with 2 tbsp granola-style cereal.

Cereal and fruit 1 bowl, 40g (1½oz) wholegrain cereal (like bran flakes, Oats 'n' More or Oatibix Flakes) topped with 1 tbsp flaked almonds, 3 or 4 dried apricots, and 125ml (4fl oz) skimmed milk.

Porridge with apples and pecan nuts Prepare 1 sachet Oat So Simple (instant porridge) according to the pack instructions. Stir in 1 tbsp chopped pecan nuts and 1 small chopped apple. Serve with extra skimmed milk.

Fruit and cheese Slice 1 medium apple and serve with 25g (1oz) reduced-fat Cheddar cheese and 10 almonds.

Grab-and-go breakfasts

Smoothie In a blender, combine a banana or a handful of frozen berries (any variety), 125ml (4fl oz) skimmed milk, 125ml (4fl oz) orange juice and 2 tbsp porridge oats. Pour into a travel cup.

Peanut butter and banana sandwich Spread 1 slice wholemeal bread with 1½ tbsp peanut butter, then add slices from ½ banana. Drizzle with 1 tsp honey and fold in half.

Wrap it Scramble 1 egg and arrange on a wholemeal tortilla. Microwave 1 slice lean back bacon for 1 minute on full power. Chop, then add to the tortilla with a handful of baby spinach. Roll up the tortilla.

Fact or fiction?

✘ FICTION: Skipping breakfast will help you lose weight.

✔ FACT: Not eating meals can lead to weight gain.

A recent British study that tracked 6,764 people found that breakfast-skippers gained twice as much weight over the course of four years as breakfast-eaters. Another research group analysed government data on 4,200 adults. They found that women who ate breakfast tended to eat fewer calories over the course of a day.

Cheese and Marmite sandwich Spread 2 slices of wholemeal bread with a little butter and Marmite, and layer with 1 tbsp grated cheese.

Breakfasts out and about

Camper's delight Munch on ¼ cup trail mix (raisins, nuts, sunflower seeds) and sip a 250ml (9fl oz) cup prepared instant hot chocolate.

Fruit smoothie 1 Innocent pomegranate, blueberry and acai smoothie, 250ml (9fl oz), plus 1 Activia strawberry yogurt.

Bar breakfast Pair a Jordan's Frusli bar with a banana and a 200ml bottle of flavoured skimmed milk.

Crunchy fruit creation Stir 1 small handful, 25g (1oz), of almonds into a 200g pack of Waitrose prepared fruit – papaya, mango and lime (or other variety or prepared fruit).

Or try these:

- 1 Caffè Nero ham and free-range egg mayonnaise breakfast muffin.
- 1 Pret A Manger bircher muesli bowl.
- 1 M & S hot porridge (plain).
- 1 McDonald's toasted bagel with 1 portion, 35g (1¼oz), Philadelphia Light cream cheese.
- 1 Starbucks breakfast pot (yogurt, apple, oats and berries) with 1 tall skinny cappuccino.
- 2 Starbucks buttermilk pancakes with 1 pack Very Berry compote.
- 1 Costa honey and granola yogurt, plus 1 pot tropical fruit sticks.
- 1 Quaker Oat So Simple express pot, sweet cinnamon flavour (add water).

Heading out for lunch? It's not easy to spot the figure-friendly options just by their names. Healthy-sounding sandwiches are often loaded with fat and calories, so look for the lower-calorie sarnies when you're shopping.

Caffè Nero
Swap 471 calories for a BLT sandwich
For 272 calories for a chicken salad sandwich
You save 199 calories

Pret A Manger
Swap 491 calories for a coronation chicken sandwich
For 373 calories for a wild crayfish and rocket sandwich
You save 118 calories

Tesco
Swap 505 calories for a red Cheddar and tomato sandwich
For 390 calories for a tuna and cucumber sandwich
You save 115 calories

Greggs
Swap 540 calories for a chicken mango bloomer
For 390 calories for Mexican chicken oval bites
You save 150 calories

Subway
Swap 368 calories for a Subway melt
For 223 calories for a 6-inch low-fat veggie delite sub
You save 145 calories

McDonald's
Swap 620 calories for a crispy chicken and bacon sandwich
For 385 calories for a McChicken sandwich
You save 235 calories

Starbucks
Swap 520 calories for a meatball panini
For 374 calories for a roasted chicken and tomato panini
You save 146 calories

Costa
Swap 520 calories for a Brie, bacon and onion chutney panini
For 423 calories for a goat's cheese and caramelized onion chutney panini
You save 97 calories: the perfect lunch to help you Drop a Dress Size!

Simple swaps

Swap this
90 calories per 250ml (9fl oz) glass orange juice
For this
60 calories per whole orange

It's easy to believe that short walks don't make a difference, but a five-minute walk, six times a day, burns off about 100 calories – which translates into 4.5kg (10lb) shed in a year. Here's how to get those six walks.

1 Park and walk
Park your car farther away from your workplace.

2 Jump off early
If you take the bus, get off a few stops early and walk the rest of the way to work.

3 Break it up
Take several five-minute walking breaks during the day. Walk around the school (teachers), the store (retail workers), the floor (office employees), or the neighbourhood (if you work from home).

4 Stretch it out
Stretch or do light strengthening exercises at your desk.

5 Meetings on the go
Hold walking meetings outdoors (you can talk and walk!).

BURN, BABY, BURN
Activity step aerobics* – with a 15–20.5cm (6–8in) step, time 30 minutes: You burn 284 calories. *Based on a 63kg (10 stone) woman. Try it in your lunch break!

6 Take the long road
Take the long route every time you go to the copy machine, a colleague's office, a classroom, etc.

7 Multitask
Sit on a stability/Swiss ball at your desk for an hour or two every day.

8 Walkie-talkie
Walk around or pace while talking on the phone.

9 Recharge your batteries
Enjoy a spot of window shopping at lunchtime.

10 Lift off
Wherever possible, opt for the stairs instead of the lift.

Choosing to take a meal to work provides a nutritious and healthy alternative to café fare and saves you money. Each of these options adds up to about 500 calories.

Take your own packed lunch

Mediterranean sandwich Spread two slices of wholemeal bread with 2 tsp pesto. Lay thin slices of mozzarella on one side of the bread, layer with thin tomato slices, halved pitted black olives and roughly chopped Cooks&Co roasted red peppers (available from Waitrose). Serve with 1 nectarine or peach. (470 calories.)

Soup lunch A flask of hot vegetable soup can provide a portion (or two) of your five-a-day and boost your fibre intake. Alternatively, warm a carton of New Covent Garden carrot and coriander soup and serve with 1 wholemeal roll, 10g (¼oz) butter and 1 clementine. (420 calories.)

Pasta box Cook 50g (2oz) pasta shapes according to the pack instructions (or use leftover cooked pasta). Combine with ½ chopped pepper, 1 chopped spring onion, 2 tbsp canned red kidney beans, 1 cooked and shredded skinless chicken breast, 1 chopped tomato, ½ sliced apple and 1 tbsp low-fat mayonnaise. Pack into a plastic box. (425 calories.)

Hummus and vegetables Have ¼ pot, 50g (2oz), low-fat hummus with 4 Nairn's oatcakes and lots of vegetable sticks (ready-prepared carrot or cucumber batons, sliced peppers, cherry tomatoes, celery and radishes). Follow with 1 Activia creamy strawberry yogurt. (450 calories.)

Diet trap

MISTAKING THIRST FOR HUNGER
That afternoon stomach pang or feeling of fatigue may be your body's way of asking for a glass of water, not a bag of crisps. How can you tell? When you feel the urge to eat, start by drinking a cup or two of water (or another zero-calorie drink) and see how you feel in five minutes' time.

 ### Step on it!

Be proactive
If your workplace cafeteria doesn't offer healthy choices, find out who's in charge of the food service and lobby for better options. Ask your manager to arrange for health professionals (nutritionists, fitness experts and so on) to speak to employees over lunch. Start a walking group at work. Take personal responsibility for your weight-loss goals and help make your workplace as healthy as possible.

Desktop dining

Each of the following meals contains about 500 calories:

- 1 Innocent Indian vegetable masala vegetable pot. Follow with 1 Müller Light strawberry yogurt.
- 1 Innocent Mexican sweet potato chilli vegetable pot. Follow with 200g (7oz) prepared pineapple.
- 1 Waitrose four-bean and wheat berry salad. Follow with 1 Waitrose LoveLife You Count probiotic cherry yogurt.
- 1 Sainsbury's giant couscous and feta salad. Follow with 150g (5oz) grapes.
- 1 Asda prawn layered pasta salad. Follow with 2 satsumas.
- 1 Tesco chargrilled chicken pasta snack salad. Follow with 1 apple.
- 1 Waitrose LoveLife You Count spiced king prawn noodle salad. Follow with Yeo Valley organic strawberry yogurt pot.
- 1 Boots Shapers around the world Japanese-style sushi. Follow with 1 banana and Boots Shapers mango chunks.

Working on the road

Business travel doesn't have to derail your Drop a Dress Size efforts. Just put these fitness tips into practice when work travel disrupts your usual routine:

If the hotel doesn't have a gym, you can turn your room into one. Pack resistance bands and a skipping rope, and use filled water bottles as substitutes for light weights. You don't need fancy equipment for push-ups, sit-ups, lunges or triceps dips (use a chair). If you travel with your laptop or smartphone, you can even go online to sites for videos of guided workouts. It's like having your own personal trainer in your hotel room!

 Step on it!

Hydrate up high

If you go on business trips that requiring flying, remember that a pressurized plane paired with salty snacks is dehydrating. When the drinks trolley rolls along, stick with water or low-cal drinks and steer clear of high-calorie fizzy drinks and juices.

Snacks in 100-calorie portions are handy for keeping in your bag, desk drawer or fridge at work. But some are healthier than others. The following ten snacks will help you stay on track with your healthy-eating intentions.

- 1 bag Cathedral City Chedds Nibbles (75 calories per 18g bag). Provides protein and calcium to help maintain strong bones.
- 1 Yeo Valley organic Yeo smoothie (97 calories per 90g pot). A mixture of yogurt and fruit purée provides protein, calcium and vitamins.
- 1 bag Nākd cherry-infused raisins (75 calories per 25g bag). These convenient packs of raisins taste like cherries and will satisfy your sweet cravings as well as providing fibre.
- 1 pot Hartley's pineapple in jelly (100 calories per 175g pot). This fat-free snack is perfect if you have a sweet tooth.
- 1 Weetabix milk chocolate oaty bar (79 calories per 23g bar). These handy bars, made with whole oats, are high in fibre and so will help stave off hunger.

- 1 Starbucks fruit salad (95 calories per pot). A super-convenient way of getting one of your five-a-day portions, this high-fibre snack is filling and full of vitamins.
- 1 Danone Actimel raspberry drinking yogurt (75 calories per 100g bottle). This low-fat drinking yogurt contains probiotics to give your immune system a boost.
- 1 bag of Twiglets (97 calories per 24g bag). A healthy alternative to crisps, Twiglets are made with whole wheat and provide 3g fibre per bag.
- 1 bag Kellogg's Special K mini breaks original (99 calories per 24g bag). A low-fat snack made from oats, wheat and rice, which won't break the calorie bank.
- 1 Waitrose LoveLife country vegetable cup soup (59 calories per sachet). This tasty soup-in-a-cup is great on a chilly day.

Diet trap

EATING WHEN YOU ARE BORED
The tedium of waiting for a delayed flight or a long journey can drive you to snack. So make sure you keep your brain active – with a book, magazine, crossword puzzle, Sudoku or MP3 player. You won't even notice you're surrounded by unhealthy foods if you're engrossed in a good film or novel.

MEAL MEMORIES

To curb late afternoon snack attacks, think about lunch. In a recent study, British researchers fed 47 women a midday meal and then, three hours later, asked them to write about either the meal or their morning commute. Those who described lunch downed one-third fewer goodies later in the day than those who recalled their travel routine. Why? Remembering your last meal helps to activate your body's natural 'I'm satisfied' signal, say researchers, so that you eat less overall.

Can't get away from the office to go to the gym? Don't worry – these simple exercises can be done at your desk (or nearby) and will help you to keep in shape at work.

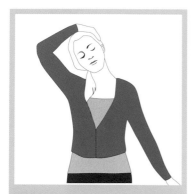

Neck roll

Tilt your head so that your right ear nearly touches your right shoulder. Using your hand, press your head a little lower (gently). Hold for 10 seconds. Relax and then repeat on the other side.

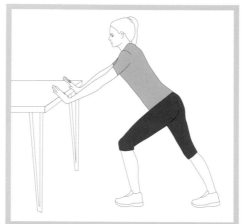

Calf stretch

From a standing position, take an exaggerated step forwards, keeping your back leg straight. Hold on to your desk for support. Your front knee should be at 90° and positioned above your foot. Lean forwards slightly so that your back leg and body make a continuous line. Hold for 15–30 seconds.

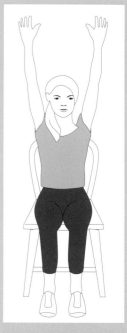

Shoulder stretch

Sitting tall in your chair, stretch both arms over your head and reach up. Hold for 10 seconds and then relax. Repeat.

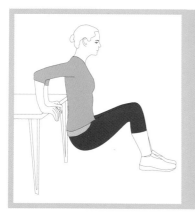

Desk dips

With your back to a desk, place your hands shoulder-width apart on the desk, fingers facing forwards. Bend your elbows and lower your body until your elbows form an angle of 90°. Hold for 2 seconds, then straighten your arms to bring you back to the starting position. Repeat 10–12 times.

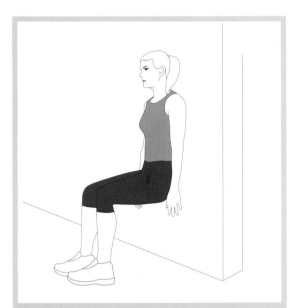

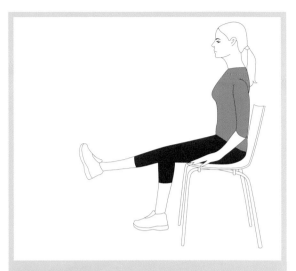

Wall slide

Lean against a wall with your feet about 30.5cm (12in) in front of you, positioned shoulder-width apart. Keeping your back flat against the wall, slowly bend your knees and lower yourself down until your knees reach a 90° bend. Hold for a second and then return to your starting position without arching your back. Repeat 10–12 times.

Leg extensions

Sitting in a chair, extend one leg out straight. Hold for a second, then lower your leg back down. Repeat 10–12 times with each leg.

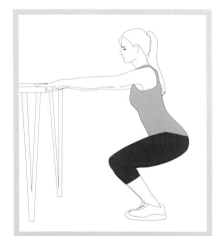

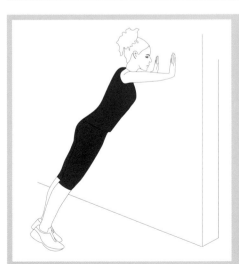

Wall press-ups

Stand about 90cm (36in) away from a wall with feet hip-width apart. Place your hands on the wall at chest height, then bend your elbows out to the side and lean in against the wall. Straighten your arms and repeat 10–12 times.

Desk squat

Face your desk and place your palms on the desktop. Squat down until your thighs are parallel to the floor. Keep your back straight and return to standing. Repeat 10–12 times.

FAT-BUSTING WEEKDAY MEAL PLANNER

	MONDAY	TUESDAY	WEDNESDAY	THURSDAY	FRIDAY
BREAKFAST (about 350 calories)	40g (1½oz) bran flakes with 2 tbsp flaked almonds, 75g (3oz) berries, and 125ml (4fl oz) skimmed milk	1 x 125ml pot Activia yogurt; 1 banana; 1 Oat So Simple morning bar	1 pot Oat So Simple; 1 tbsp nuts and 2 tbsp raisins	2 slices of wholemeal bread spread with a little butter and Marmite, 1 tbsp grated cheese	1 Innocent blackberry, strawberry and blackcurrant smoothie, 250ml, plus 1 x 170ml pot Total fat-free Greek yogurt with honey
LUNCH (about 500 calories)	1 carton New Covent Garden tomato and basil soup; 1 wholemeal roll with 10g (¼oz) butter; 1 clementine	1 Innocent Mexican sweet potato chilli vegetable pot; 200g (7oz) prepared pineapple	4 Nairn's oatcakes, ¼ pot, 50g (2oz), low-fat hummus, veg sticks; 1 x 125ml pot Activia yogurt	1 Sainsbury's giant couscous and feta salad; 150g (5oz) grapes	1 Caffè Nero chicken salad sandwich; 1 nectarine; 1 grande Caffè Nero latte (skimmed milk)
DINNER (about 500 calories)	Grilled Spicy Chicken (p. 130); 4 tbsp cooked wholegrain rice; broccoli; 80g (3¼oz) berries with 1 tbsp fat Greek yogurt	Cod with Cherry Tomatoes (p. 131); 175g (6oz) baked potato, 2 tsp butter; 150g (5oz) fruit salad, 1 tbsp fat-free Greek yogurt	Spiced Lamb with Lentils (p. 140); 150g (5oz) new potatoes; leafy salad; 125g (4oz) berries	Thai Vegetable Curry (p. 136) with 4 tbsp cooked wholegrain rice; 1 x 125g pot low-fat yogurt	Classic Lasagne (p. 132) with carrots and green beans; 125g (4oz) fresh fruit
SNACK (about 100 calories)	1 x 125g Müller Vitality yogurt (any)	20g (¾oz) mixed nuts	1 Weetabix oaty bar (any flavour)	2 rice cakes; 1 satsuma	1 banana

Find which eating type you conform to in the workplace, then learn tricks to eat better.

STYLE	BEHAVIOUR	TIPS
GRAZER	You can't walk through the canteen without grabbing a doughnut or a Danish, or you regularly pick up treats in the office kitchen. You often snack out of habit, not hunger.	Keep low-cal, nutritious items such as grapes, baby carrots and berries at hand so you can graze without the damage. Eat only in designated areas (in the lunch room, for example) – not in meeting rooms or at your desk.
STUFFER	You have what grandmas call a 'healthy appetite'. Although you rarely snack in the office, at mealtimes you clean your plate and often go for seconds.	Instead of eating until you're stuffed, tune in to your body for cues that tell you you're no longer hungry – it takes practice to become more aware.
PARTY BINGER	You're good at watching your food choices, except at office social events. At colleagues' birthday parties and clients' events, for example, you pay no attention to how much you're consuming.	Chew sugar-free gum or mints at events to keep your mouth occupied and as a reminder to watch what you eat. When you're chatting with someone, set your food aside. If you don't, you could eat every bite without tasting any of it.

Eating out

Eating away from home doesn't have to spell trouble for your calorie bottom line. We show you how to keep your waistline in mind, whether you're grabbing fast food or visiting your favourite restaurant.

When you eat out, your good intentions often fly out of the window. After all, it's easy to relax and overindulge when someone else is doing the cooking – and the dishes! Plus, restaurant meals have a lot more calories at least 60 per cent more, according to one recent study) than the same dishes prepared at home.

A meal out used to be a special occasion, but in today's fast-paced world, in which we're all juggling busy careers, family responsibilities and social commitments, eating out is more likely to be a time (and sanity) saving strategy. In fact, the average person eats about five meals outside the home each week; however, there's always a healthy choice you can make, whether you're at a coffee chain or a family restaurant.

1 Get in the know

When the California Center for Public Health Advocacy recently asked 523 people to name the healthiest options at popular restaurants, 68 per cent didn't get a single answer right. Guesstimating nutrition information just doesn't work. Do yourself a favour, and do a little research. Many restaurants post their entire menu plus nutrition information online, making it easy for you to make informed choices ahead of time, so if, like most people, you tend to frequent the same spots over and over again, go online or ask for in-house nutrition leaflets, and find healthy options at your five favourites.

It's always a good idea to make healthy out-and-about options (that is, nutrient-rich meals packed with filling fibre and low in saturated fat, refined sugars and salt), but when you are trying to drop pounds, calories are what count. And keeping your overall calorie intake in mind gives you the freedom to make a less than ideal choice once in a while.

2 Eat consciously

People who manage to lose weight are aware of just how much they eat and drink, and when they overindulge occasionally they'll make up for it later (see Practise Damage Control opposite). People who struggle with their weight, however, tend to ignore their body's cues and often eat past the point of fullness. It's easy to get sucked into overeating: researchers at Cornell University hosted a Super Bowl party for 50 people and served an unlimited number of chicken wings. At half the tables, waiters scooped away the bones as they ate. At the other tables, where party-goers could see their scraps piling up, they ate 27 per cent less.

When you are dining out, it's extra important to pay attention to what your body is telling you, since portions are often oversized. As soon as you start to feel full, put down your fork, spoon, pastry or sandwich – stop eating, and give yourself a few minutes to check your hunger before you eat more. Clean plates are not required.

3 Manage your hunger

When you skip meals or go hungry in order to save calories for a lunch out or a social function later in the day, you set yourself up for a dining-out disaster. You'll be so ravenous by the time you get to your dinner, party or event that you'll end up eating a lot more than if you had eaten a healthy meal earlier in the day. What's more, skipping meals can result in a slowed

Diet trap

CRAVING JUNK?

Scientists in the US have discovered why many dieters start craving junk foods. It's all to do with the speed of weight loss. Dropping weight too quickly increases your stress levels, making dieting more difficult and reprogramming the way the brain deals with future stressful situations. This means that when you are put under stress, you are more likely to reach for fatty and sugary foods, the very foods you denied yourself while dieting. So if you need to lose a few pounds:
• Aim to lose weight gradually: no more than 1kg (2¼lb) per week.
• Don't ban your favourite foods. Little treats are fine – studies show that your taste buds are satisfied after the first three or four bites.

metabolism as your 'starving' body assumes you are in a state of emergency and starts conserving fat. Keeping yourself satisfied over the course of the day helps to maintain your appetite (and your metabolism) on an even keel, giving you a much better chance to eat consciously, make better choices and actually enjoy your meals.

4 Find a balance

You've heard it before, but lots of restaurant foods are full of fat and calories. Some of the worst offenders are cream, cheese, ice cream, butter, puddings, fried foods and fatty meats. So how do you make smarter choices? Look for foods that are most like their natural state – fruits, vegetables, beans and whole grains, rather than burgers, chips or fruit pies. The better options will contain more vitamins, minerals, antioxidants, phytochemicals and filling fibre.

Research shows that people who completely ban their favourite foods while trying to lose weight tend to cycle between dieting and bingeing on the foods they restrict. Balancing choices is key. So, if breakfast out is just not the same without a few rashers of bacon, have them with a slice of wholegrain toast and fresh fruit. If you can't live without the chips or sautéed potatoes at your favourite restaurant, order grilled fish and vegetables as your main course and share the fries with your dining companion. If you are craving a decadent dessert, share it with a friend (or two or three).

5 Practise damage control

In the real world of dining out and dieting, making the best choices, eating consciously, finding a balance or just saying no (to the bread basket, French fries, dessert or a second glass of wine) is not always possible. If you occasionally have an indulgent meal – you know it happens – and you still want to Drop a Dress Size, you have to be prepared to neutralize the damage. Choose lower-calorie options for your next few meals and increase your activity level for several days, and your indulgence won't have a chance to stick to your hips (or bottom or stomach).

PRACTISE PORTION CONTROL

When you are trying to Drop a Dress Size, portion control is key. Use the visual clues below to help you avoid portion distortion while dining out. If you are served too much (which is likely), share it or take some home.

75g (3oz) portion of fish, poultry or meat: lean protein is a good choice for dieters, so it's OK to double this serving size to 175g (6oz):
THE SIZE OF AN IPHONE

25g (1oz) portion of cheese or chocolate:
THE SIZE OF ABOUT 4 DICE

2 tbsp portion of dressing:
THE AMOUNT IN A SHOT GLASS

100g (3½oz) portion of grains, rice, pasta or ice cream:
THE SIZE OF A TENNIS BALL

1 tsp portion of butter or margarine:
THE SIZE OF A SCRABBLE TILE

Small bread roll:
THE SIZE OF A COMPUTER MOUSE

Handful of dried fruit or nuts:
THE SIZE OF 1 LARGE EGG

Average bagel:
THE SIZE OF A 12.5CM (5IN) ROUND MAKE-UP COMPACT

Medium potato:
THE SIZE OF A TENNIS BALL

Diet trap

SUPER-SIZING
A study at Penn State University found that super-sized restaurant portions result in a higher calorie intake. The size of a pasta dish was varied between a standard portion and a portion 50 per cent larger. Those who were served the bigger portion ate nearly all of it – consuming an extra 172 calories. But all customers rated the size of both portions equally appropriate for meeting their needs. So, if you don't want to eat more than you need, steer clear of super-sizing.

Did you know?

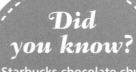

1 Starbucks chocolate chunk cookie = 8½ Maryland chocolate chip cookies = 499 calories.

Simple eating-out swaps

Save at least 100 calories with each of these restaurant and takeaway swaps:

Swap 550 calories for 200g (7oz) crispy king prawns with 200g (7oz) egg-fried rice
For 360 calories for a 400g (14oz) portion of chicken chow mein
You save 190 calories

Swap 422 calories for 1 Costa banana and pecan breakfast loaf
For 276 calories for 1 Costa butter croissant
You save 146 calories

Swap 191 calories for 1 Millie's white chocolate cookie
For 80 calories for 1 Cadbury's oat and chocolate chip cookie
You save 111 calories

Swap 223 calories for Yo Sushi! salmon teriyaki
For 99 calories Yo Sushi! crispy salmon skin hand roll
You save 124 calories

Swap 482 calories for a slice of Starbucks blueberry cheesecake
For 348 calories for a Starbucks granola bar
You save 134 calories

Swap 238 calories for a Starbucks grande frappuccino
For 126 calories for a Starbucks grande iced caffè latte made with semi-skimmed milk
You save 112 calories

Swap 350 calories for 1 portion of Pizza Express dough balls with butter
For 246 calories for 1 portion of Pizza Express garlic bread
You save 104 calories

If you're out and about, you don't have to derail your diet. Here are the options that spell trouble – and what to get instead.

BREAKFAST			
DIET MADNESS	DIET MAKEOVER	YOU SAVE	SWAP ONCE A WEEK
Starbucks: 1 bacon butty with a grande latte *637 calories*	Starbucks: 2 buttermilk pancakes with Very Berry compote; 1 grande caffè Americano *303 calories*	*334 calories*	Drop 450g/0.5kg (1lb) in 10½ weeks
McDonald's: 1 sausage and egg McMuffin; cappuccino *550 calories*	McDonald's: 1 Oat So Simple porridge with a regular coffee *225 calories*	*325 calories*	Drop 450g/0.5kg (1lb) in 10½ weeks
Costa: 1 all-day breakfast roll with a flat white coffee *798 calories*	Costa: 1 strawberry granola yogurt with a Costa light coffee *341 calories*	*457 calories*	Drop 450g/0.5kg (1lb) in 8 weeks

SNACK			
DIET MADNESS	DIET MAKEOVER	YOU SAVE	SWAP TWICE A WEEK
Caffè Nero: 1 blueberry muffin *438 calories*	Caffè Nero: 1 almond biscotti *147 calories*	*291 calories*	Drop 450g/0.5kg (1lb) in 12 weeks
Costa: 1 carrot cake *514 calories*	Costa : 1 mini chocolate muffin *73 calories*	*441 calories*	Drop 450g/0.5kg (1lb) in 8 weeks
M & S Café: fruit scone with butter, jam and clotted cream *645 calories*	M & S Café: 2 shortbreads *206 calories*	*439 calories*	Drop 450g/0.5kg (1lb) In 8 weeks

LUNCH/DINNER

DIET MADNESS	DIET MAKEOVER	YOU SAVE	SWAP TWICE A WEEK
Caffè Nero: 1 BLT sandwich 471 calories	Caffè Nero: 1 mozzarella and cherry tomato salad 276 calories	195 calories	Drop 450g/0.5kg (1lb) in 18 weeks
Starbucks: 1 tuna melt and mature cheese panini; 1 packet sea salt crisps 737 calories	Starbucks: 1 roasted chicken salsa wrap; 1 fruit salad pot 482 calories	255 calories	Drop 450g/0.5kg (1lb) in 14 weeks
Pizza Express: 1 fiorentina classic pizza 809 calories	Pizza Express: 1 pomodoro pesto leggera pizza 500 calories	309 calories	Drop 450g/0.5kg (1lb) in 11½ weeks
Prezzo: 1 serving crab cakes and courgette fries 1,265 calories	Prezzo: 1 pollo Siciliana and gratinated potatoes 498 calories	767 calories	Drop 450g/0.5kg (1lb) in 5 weeks
JD Wetherspoon: 1 x 8oz sirloin steak with chips, peas and tomato 987 calories	JD Wetherspoon: 1 chicken breast and pepper skewers with piri-piri sauce 449 calories	538 calories	Drop 450g/0.5kg (1lb) in 6½ weeks
Pizza Hut: 1 regular, 23cm (9in), chicken supreme pan pizza 1,038 calories	Pizza Hut: 1 virtuous veg pizzetta 439 calories	599 calories	Drop 450g/0.5kg (1lb) in 6 weeks
Harvester: 1 gammon steak with pineapple, fries and gravy 1,340 calories	Harvester: 2 piri-piri chicken skewers, baby potatoes and hot piri-piri sauce 500 calories	840 calories	Drop 450g/0.5kg (1lb) in 4½ weeks
Pret A Manger: 1 Brie and bacon artisan baguette 653 calories	Pret A Manger: 1 veggie sushi 333 calories	320 calories	Drop 450g/0.5kg (1lb) in 11 weeks

Eating on the run doesn't have to spell diet disaster. Here's a cheat sheet to help you avoid major calorie pitfalls – and what to order instead.

McDonald's

SWAP	FOR	YOU SAVE
1 cheeseburger with medium fries *625 calories*	1 grilled chicken salad wrap; fruit bag *372 calories*	*253 calories*
1 Big Mac with medium fries *820 calories*	1 grilled chicken salad; iced mango and pineapple smoothie *305 calories*	*515 calories*
1 chicken legend with medium fries *880 calories*	1 hamburger with a garden side salad (without dressing) *260 calories*	*620 calories*
1 crispy chicken and bacon wrap; strawberry shake *875 calories*	1 spicy veggie wrap with carrot sticks *449 calories*	*426 calories*

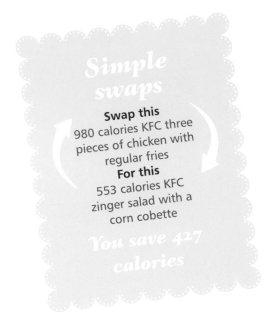

Simple swaps

Swap this
980 calories KFC three pieces of chicken with regular fries
For this
553 calories KFC zinger salad with a corn cobette

You save 427 calories

Spudulike toppings

SWAP	FOR	YOU SAVE
Chicken tikka *233 calories*	Baked beans *69 calories*	*164 calories*
Coleslaw *190 calories*	Cottage cheese *84 calories*	*106 calories*
Grated cheese *250 calories*	Chilli con carne *101 calories*	*149 calories*

Wimpy

SWAP	FOR	YOU SAVE
1 hamburger and cheese with chips 846 *calories*	1 chicken fillet burger 356 *calories*	490 *calories*
1 Wimpy grill 757 *calories*	1 Wimpy hamburger 330 *calories*	427 *calories*
1 spicy bean burger with chips 878 *calories*	1 jacket potato with butter and salad 453 *calories*	425 *calories*

Swap this
689 calories for a Nando's double chicken breast fillet wrap
For this
347 calories for a Nando's chicken breast in pitta

Burger King

SWAP	FOR	YOU SAVE
1 Whopper with regular fries 942 *calories*	1 sweet chilli chicken wrap with a garden salad 329 *calories*	613 *calories*
1 chicken royale; large coke 860 *calories*	1 flame-grilled chicken salad; Tropicana orange juice 246 *calories*	614 *calories*
1 smoked bacon and Cheddar Angus burger with regular fries 991 *calories*	1 ocean catch 493 *calories*	498 *calories*
1 chicken tendercrisp; regular chocolate shake 1,085 *calories*	1 veggie wrap 459 *calories*	626 *calories*

High-calorie, oil-laden salad bar choices abound, but stick to our top ten list and you'll find it easy to build a winning weight-loss salad.

1 Leafy greens

Why? Skip nutrient-poor, boring iceberg lettuce and load up on tastier and healthier leaves, including baby spinach, watercress and mixed leaves.

How much? The sky's the limit.

2 Beans

Why? Loaded with protein, fibre and nutrients, beans make you feel fuller faster and stay full for longer. Chickpeas and red kidney beans are the types most commonly found in salad bars.

How much? About 2 tbsp: 40 calories.

3 Fresh vegetables

Why? Low in calories but high in nutrients and fibre. Go for undressed options (broccoli, tomatoes, green beans, carrots) with lots of colour and variety, and steer clear of calorie-laden dressed vegetable salads such as coleslaw and potato salad.

How much? Keep calorie-dense, starchy vegetables (such as sweetcorn and potatoes) to about 1 tbsp: 30 calories; otherwise, there's no limit.

4 Fresh fruit

Why? Fruit is low in calories and supplies not just tangy flavour but also phytochemicals, vitamins, minerals and fibre.

How much? About 2 tbsp: 20–60 calories.

5 Nuts and seeds

Why? Packed with protein and nutrients, nuts and seeds add a wholesome crunch.

How much? Limit to 1 tbsp to keep calories in check: 45 calories.

6 Cheese

Why? To increase salad satisfaction, choose a strong-flavoured full-fat cheese (such as grated Parmesan or crumbled feta or blue cheese), but use it sparingly.

How much? About 1 tbsp grated cheese: 25 calories.

7 Olives

Why? Rich in heart-healthy monounsaturated fats and flavour.

How much? A little goes a long way, so limit this calorie-dense option to about 2 tbsp sliced or 3 or 4 whole olives: 30 calories.

8 Hard-boiled eggs

Why? Lots of protein, 6g (¼oz) per egg, nutrients and flavour.

How much? About 2 tbsp chopped egg or ½ egg: 30 calories.

9 Grilled skinless chicken

Why? A low-calorie, protein-rich choice to help you feel full for longer.

How much? About 2 tbsp, chopped: 60 calories.

10 Light dressing

Why? Full-fat dressings can ruin a perfectly good Drop a Dress Size salad by adding hundreds of unwanted calories; light versions add flavour with minimal calorie impact.

How much? 2 tbsp: 50–80 calories.

Know your dressings

	Average portion	Calories	Fat (g)	Saturated fat (g)
Barbecue sauce	20g (1 tbsp)	19	0	0
Branston pickle, Crosse & Blackwell	30g (1 tbsp)	33	0.1	0
Brown sauce	20g (1 tbsp)	20	0	0
Chilli sauce	20g (1 tbsp)	16	0	0
French dressing	15g (1 tbsp)	98	11	1.5
Horseradish sauce	20g (1 tbsp)	31	2	0.2
Light mayonnaise, Hellman's	30g (1 tbsp)	88	8.9	0.9
Mango chutney	30g (1 tbsp)	57	0	0
Mayonnaise	30g (1 tbsp)	207	23	3.4
Salad cream	20g (1 tbsp)	70	6	0.7
Soy sauce	15g (1 tbsp)	10	0	0

 Step on it!

Start with salad
A Penn State University study found that women who had a salad starter (without dressing) before a pasta lunch ate fewer calories over the course of a meal than those who dug straight into the carbs.

You can still eat out in your favourite restaurants but careful selection is key if you want to stay within your Drop a Dress Size guidelines.

Step on it!

Clue into keywords on the menu
Words such as 'battered' or 'crispy' usually mean the items are fried, while 'au gratin', 'creamed' and 'scalloped' indicate they're loaded with cream or cheese – or both (all translate to lots of calories and fat). Terms such as 'grilled', 'baked' or 'steamed' tend to indicate healthier and lower-calorie options.

Chinese

Food from a Chinese restaurant is loaded with lots of good-for-your-waist (and heart) options if you choose carefully. Look for dishes with vegetables, seafood, tofu or poultry as the star players. Also, order steamed rice (brown rice, if you can find it) instead of fried rice or noodles.

Limit battered, breaded or fried items. In Chinese food lingo, 'crispy' equals 'fried'. Even tofu can turn into a no-no after a turn in the deep-fryer. Also, be wary about dishes made with nuts. Although they're healthy, too many nuts make for too many calories. Mix your main course with a portion of steamed vegetables to turn it into a lower-calorie and lower-fat meal. In general, stick with half a portion of a dish mixed with one portion of steamed vegetables served with half a portion of rice.

Mix and match the Japanese menu items opposite for a healthy lunch.

Japanese restaurant	
Roll (1)	**Calories**
Avocado roll	140
California roll	255
Cucumber roll	135
Eel and avocado roll	370
Salmon and avocado roll	305
Shrimp tempura roll	510
Spicy tuna roll	290
Sushi (1 piece)	
Abalone	45
Bonito	45
Eel	65
Flounder	45
Giant scallop	45
Salmon	50
Shrimp	60
Squid	45
Tuna (bluefin)	50
White tuna (albacore)	55
Whiting	40
Yellowtail	50
Other	
Edamame beans	100
Miso soup	40
Soy sauce (1 tsp)	10

Indian

Remember to avoid the rich sauces. Thumbs up to dishes such as chicken tikka, channa dhal (chickpeas), dhal (lentils), and vegetable side dishes offer diners plenty of delicious ways to enjoy Indian food while you Drop a Dress Size. Bhuna, dupiaza, vindaloo and Madras dishes are likely to be lower in fat than those in rich sauces. Opt for a plain chapatti made without fat – you'll save 10g (¼oz) fat and 130 calories compared with a naan bread, which contains fat. Naan bread can pack up to 540 calories into a portion, so limit yourself to a quarter-portion, or simply skip it altogether.

Thumbs down to chicken tikka masala, rogan josh, biryanis and jaipuris, and anything in a korma, passanda or masala sauce. All spell big trouble for your waist and heart, delivering up to 800 calories per portion.

Italian

Look for the delicious and nutritious low-fat options below and you can enjoy the taste of the Mediterranean without the guilt.

Italian restaurant

PICK	PASS ON
PASTA	
Pasta paired with red sauces (such as marinara and other tomato sauces), clam sauce, vegetables (like pasta primavera made with olive oil, not cream), and grilled chicken or seafood.	Pasta paired with cream, cheese or butter sauces (like Alfredo and carbonara), meat (such as meatballs or sausage), and sauces made with meat (such as bolognese).
PIZZA	
Thin-crust or small-sized pizzas with lots of vegetables, less cheese (or, even better, no cheese), lean meat (like ham or chicken) and, when available, a healthier wholemeal crust.	Deep-dish pizzas with extra cheese and fatty meat toppings (like sausage, mince, pork or pepperoni) or stuffed crusts.
SALADS	
Mixed green salads loaded with fresh vegetables, with dressings and cheese on the side (and used sparingly).	Caesar salads, caprese (mozzarella and tomato) salads, and meat-and-cheese antipasti salads.
CLASSICS	
Simply prepared (steamed and grilled) fish and chicken dishes.	Parmigiana dishes (like aubergine Parmigiana), dishes loaded with cheese and meat (like manicotti and lasagne), and fried foods (like calamari fritti or mozzarella fritta).

For healthy and flavoursome sandwiches that will satisfy your hunger and keep the weight falling off, keep to a few sandwich 'rules'.

Sandwich dos

Deli sandwiches are fast and convenient, but you pay the price in fat and calories. Make your stop at the deli counter a Drop a Dress Size.

Do Order lean fillings. Roast beef, ham, turkey and chicken breasts have half (or less) the calories and fat of pepperoni, salami, bacon, salami and cheeses such as Cheddar, Brie and Stilton.

Do Pile on vegetables. Fresh (like rocket, baby spinach, tomatoes and cucumbers) and roasted (such as onions, peppers and courgette), as well as pickles, are all low-calorie choices.

Do Skip the mayo, pesto, horseradish sauce, dressings, and 'special' sauces, and opt for mustard, relish or salsa instead.

Do Get your sandwich on fibre-rich 100 per cent wholemeal or wholegrain bread (just ask the sandwich-maker). Not only is this a healthier option but the fibre is filling too.

Do Be wary of calorie-laden tuna or chicken salads made with mayonnaise; they contain 100 calories per tablespoon.

Popular sandwich choices

	CALORIES
STARBUCKS	
1 cheese and Marmite panini	382
1 mozzarella and slow-roasted tomato panini	468
1 roasted chicken and tomato panini	347
CAFFÈ NERO	
1 chicken Caesar wrap	434
1 chicken salad sandwich	272
1 falafel wrap	434
1 ham and free-range egg mayonnaise breakfast muffin	314
1 pesto chicken panini	385
1 tuna melt panini	389
1 vine tomato, mozzarella and basil panini	398

Bread basics	AVERAGE PORTION	CALORIES
Bagel, plain	85g	232
Brioche roll	35g	129
Brown bread, sliced	1 slice, 40g	85
Burger bun	85g	224
Chapatti	55g	111
Ciabatta bread	1 slice, 30g	92
Croissant	40g	186
Crumpet	40g	77
French stick	1 slice, 40g	105
Garlic bread	1 slice, 30g	110
Hovis Best of Both	1 slice, 40g	86
Hovis Seed Sensation	1 slice, 44g	122
Muffin, plain	67g	174
Naan bread	160g	456
Pitta bread, white	60g	153
Pitta bread, wholemeal	60g	159
Rye bread	1 slice, 40g	88
Scotch pancake (Kingsmill)	28g	74
Soda bread	1 slice, 40g	103
Tortilla, plain	55g	144
White bread, sliced	1 slice, 40g	88
White roll, crusty	50g	131
White roll, soft	50g	127
Wholemeal bread, sliced	1 slice, 40g	87
Wholemeal roll	50g	122
Wrap	64g	182

Fancy a burger at your favourite burger bar? There's no need to miss out. Make a slimline burger at home instead, which has all the flavour but fewer calories. You can even make healthier versions of fish and chips, or a curry, plus ice cream to follow. Staying in was never so appealing.

Slimline Burgers

Try these tasty tuna burgers instead of traditional beefburgers:

In a small bowl, stir together 1 tbsp sesame oil, 1 tbsp vegetable oil and a 2.5cm (1in) piece of fresh root ginger, grated. Brush the mixture over 4 × 125g (4oz) tuna steaks. Cook on a griddle over a high heat for 4 minutes, turning once, or for longer or shorter depending on your preference. Drizzle with a little soy sauce before serving. (Serves 4, 208 calories each.) (See also the Healthy Burger on page 20.)

Fat-free Ice Cream

Ice cream is full of fat, but you can create a fabulous alternative using frozen bananas. Here's how:

Chop 5–6 bananas and open-freeze on a baking tray until solid (about 4 hours). Tip into a food processor with 5 tbsp milk and whizz until smooth. Drizzle with a little honey, if you like, and serve. (Serves 4, 143 calories per serving.)

Low-fat Fish and Chips

Deep-fried fish and chips might be a match made in heaven, but this meal is hell in the fat stakes. Here's how to lower the fat without losing flavour:

Make chips by slicing 2 large potatoes into wedges, then put on a non-stick baking tray. Pour ½ tbsp olive oil over them, season and cook at 200°C (180°C fan oven) mark 6 for 30 minutes. For the fish, dip white fish fillets into flour, then egg, then breadcrumbs. Spray lightly with oil and grill for 4–5 minutes per side until done. (Serves 4, 364 calories per serving.)

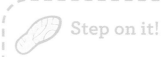 Step on it!

Track your wrappers
To prevent yourself from mindlessly munching through half a dozen bite-sized treats on the sofa, count your empty wrappers. This will help you to keep a tally of your intake and remind you to stop snacking.

Healthy Curry

Swap your usual takeaway curry for this easy-to-make vegetarian dish:

Heat 1 tbsp curry paste in a large, heavy-based pan for 1 minute, stirring the paste to warm the spices. Add a 227g can chopped tomatoes and 150ml (¼ pint) hot vegetable stock. Bring to the boil, then reduce the heat to a simmer and add 200g chopped vegetables (such as broccoli, courgettes and sugarsnap peas). Simmer for 5–6 minutes until the vegetables are tender. Stir in ½ × 400g can chickpeas and heat for 1–2 minutes. Serve with a warm wholemeal pitta bread and low-fat natural yogurt. (Serves 4, 525 calories per serving.)

Diet trap

NOT COUNTING ALCOHOL
Studies have shown that drinking one
alcoholic beverage a day could improve a
woman's heart health – but that doesn't give
you carte blanche to guzzle wine at dinner.
Once you exceed the one-drink maximum, it's
no longer heart-healthy – or diet-friendly –
to keep sipping. (To get a sense of how
quickly the calories from alcohol can
add up, consult the chart on pages
122–23.)

Here's a workout that you can do outdoors, be it in your local park or back garden. It combines aerobic moves with strengthening exercises to tone your muscles and burn calories.

Walk or jog
Warm up by walking or jogging for 2 minutes. You should feel as though you're working, but be able to carry on a conversation without huffing and puffing.

Speed-walk or jog
Speed-walk or jog for 2 minutes so that you're raising your heart rate a little more.

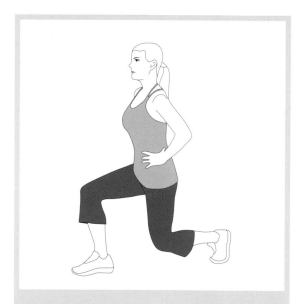

Walking lunges
Take a big step forward with the right foot and lower into a lunge (keeping the front knee behind the toe), step the left foot next to the right and then into a lunge on the left side. Repeat 10 times for each leg.

Sprints
Choose an object in the distance (a tree, a lamppost, etc.) and run or walk to it as fast as you can. Walk to recover, and repeat the sprint twice more.

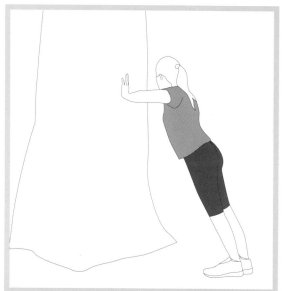

Tree push-ups
Find a tree and stand about 60–90cm (24–36in) away from it. Place your hands on the tree in front of you at about shoulder level. Bend your elbows and lean towards the tree in a push-up. Push back up, and repeat 10 times.

Speed-walk or jog
Speed walk or jog for 1 minute.

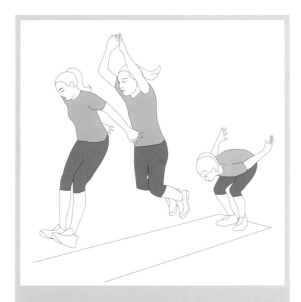

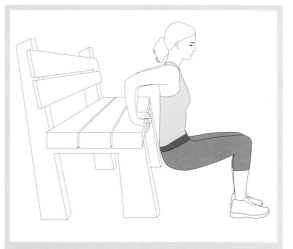

Bench dips

Sit on a bench with your hands resting on it either side of you, fingers pointing forwards. Walk your feet forwards, knees bent, and lower yourself down until your upper arms are parallel to the ground. Then push back up to straighten your arms. Repeat 10–12 times.

Long jump

Find a flat stretch of grass and begin with feet together. Lower into a slight squat and jump forward with both feet as far as you can, swinging your arms to help propel you forward. Repeat 8–10 times.

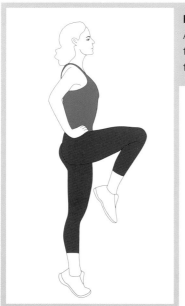

Knee-raises

As you walk or jog, lift the knees up to hip level (if you can). Do this 10 times with each leg.

Cool down

Walk for 3 minutes until your breathing rate returns to normal.

FAT-BUSTING WEEKDAY MEAL PLANNER

	MONDAY	TUESDAY	WEDNESDAY	THURSDAY	FRIDAY
BREAKFAST (about 350 calories)	40g (1½oz) Oatibix flakes with 1 sliced banana and 125ml (4fl oz) skimmed milk	2 slices of wholemeal toast with 2 tsp butter and 2 tsp honey; 1 clementine	1 Costa strawberry granola yogurt; 1 Costa light coffee	1 x 125ml pot probiotic yogurt; 1 clementine; 1 Oat So Simple morning bar	1 McDonald's Oat So Simple porridge; 1 regular coffee
LUNCH (about 500 calories)	1 Caffè Nero mozzarella and cherry tomato salad; 1 Caffè Nero bio-yogurt with honey	1 Starbucks roasted chicken salsa wrap; 1 Starbucks fruit salad pot	1 Spudulike baked potato with baked beans; 1 apple	1 Pret A Manger: veggie sushi; 1 Pret five-berry pot	1 Tesco tuna and cucumber sandwich; 1 x 200g (7oz) Tesco juicy pineapple chunks
DINNER (about 500 calories)	1 Pizza Hut virtuous veg pizzetta	120g/4¼oz grilled white fish fillet; 200g (7oz) roasted vegetables; 1 medium jacket potato with 1 tsp butter	75g (3oz) grilled pork fillet with stir-fried vegetables and 3 tbsp cooked noodles	150g (5oz) pan-fried tuna steak with spinach and 3 tbsp wholegrain cooked rice; 150g (5oz) fruit salad	1 Pizza Express pomodoro pesto leggera pizza
Snack (about 100 calories)	1 pear and 3 plums	1 Costa mini chocolate muffin	125g (4oz) grapes and 1 clementine	1 Pret A Manger fruit salad	1 x 125g pot Activia probiotic yogurt

Here are some practical strategies to help you manage portions when eating out. They will save your waistline some inches and your wallet a few pounds too!

Bigger is not better
Restaurant and fast-food portions are oversized. Don't add insult to injury by 'going large' even if it seems better value – you would be short-changing your health and your waistline. And don't be embarrassed to leave food on your plate once you've eaten enough.

Start as you mean to go on
Avoid anything bread-based for starters – dough balls, garlic bread – these are all too easy to over-consume when you're hungry. Instead, start with a simple (undressed) salad or (non-creamy) soup – both will fill you up and take the edge off your appetite.

Downsize that dinner!
Order starter-sized portions of main courses and don't be afraid to ask if you can have the lunch-sized dish at dinner time. Many restaurants offer lunch-size portions of their dishes, which are smaller than their full-sized dinner dishes. Or ask to order from the children's menu! Kids' meals contain what used to be normal-sized portions for us grown-ups.

Have a healthy snack before dining out
Avoid overeating in restaurants by not letting yourself get too hungry. Have a small, healthy snack, such as fruit or a rice cake with peanut butter, before you go out so you won't be starving when it's time to order.

Measure up carefully
While the oft-quoted small glass of red wine at 85 calories doesn't sound too ruinous, in reality most bars and restaurants serve more generous-sized measures of 175ml (6fl oz) (119 calories) and 250ml (9fl oz) (170 calories). A couple of big glasses could cost you more than the calorie equivalent of a cheeseburger (299 calories).

Slow down
Try to keep pace with the slowest eater at the table. Take time to savour the flavours of the meal and enjoy the company you are with.

In the supermarket

Supermarket shopping with your waistline in mind requires a sharp eye and willpower. What with some food manufacturers' sneaky marketing tactics, genius product placement and delicious-smelling in-store bakeries, it's easy to sabotage your diet. And since the average shopper makes two trips to the supermarket per week, that's two occasions on which you may be tempted.

These food-buying expeditions don't have to be a giant diet trap. We'll show you how to stock your kitchen with the best choices your supermarket has to offer. We've done the homework for you, scouting out the tastiest brand-name foods – from salad dressings to cheeses to frozen treats, and more – that all fit within the Drop a Dress Size calorie guidelines. Plus, our tips will help you go beyond what we've suggested to create your own list of favourite foods.

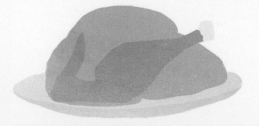

1 Stick to a list

Who would have thought that shopping with a carefully crafted shopping list could cut the amount of calories you load into your trolley by almost half? In a Lincoln University study, participants who were taught to prepare a weekly menu, convert it into a shopping list, adjust the list for foods already to hand, and organize it according to a supermarket's layout purchased about 6,500 fewer calories per week when compared to their previous trips without the menu and list-making training.

Over the remaining seven weeks of the 12-week study, the total calorie saving was nearly 46,000 calories. Better still, fewer calories in the trolley translated into weight loss – to the tune of at least 2.3kg (5lb) per person over the 12 weeks.

The key is to structure your list around a weekly menu. Set aside time before you shop to plan meals and snacks, taking into consideration your family's competing schedules and what you already have to hand. Use our recipes (see pages 128–141), the Drop a Dress Size meals throughout the book, and our Fat-Busting Weekday Meal Planners to help you create a healthy, low-cal menu and shopping list.

2 Family matters

You'll find it much easier to Drop a Dress Size (and keep the pounds off) if you and your family adopt a healthier lifestyle; however, when possible, it's best to shop for groceries alone. Not only will it speed up your trip but you will also avoid caving in on your kids' and partner's food demands. When shopping solo is not an option, find fun ways to involve your family. Plan the week's meals and shopping list together, and then tackle the supermarket as a team. Teach your kids how to read labels and encourage them to pick out new fruits, vegetables and other healthy foods for the trolley.

Don't worry: you can still include some yummy indulgences! Think moderation instead of elimination, buy calorie-controlled portions (or divvy up large bags of goodies into smaller packs when you get home), and limit treats to one per person per trip.

 Step on it!

ADD FRUIT TO YOUR CEREAL
Adding fresh berries, sliced bananas, peaches or whatever is in season to your bowl of wholegrain cereal is a wonderful way to sneak more fruit into your diet. It not only adds a sweet flavour but it also provides lots of satisfying fibre.

centre. Regularly bought items tend to be spread around the store, so we are guided past many other tempting goodies to complete our shopping. Head to the middle aisles first for things such as canned beans, wholegrain cereals and pasta – but resist going up and down all the centre aisles. Linger in the outer aisles instead, where you can pick up perishables after the packaged goods. That way, they'll stay fresher and they're less likely to get crushed.

5 Be a label spy

Just because a food is marked 'fat-free', 'sugar-free' or 'low-fat' doesn't mean it's low in calories, so be sure to carefully read the nutrition information panel. Don't forget to check the serving size, too: sometimes an item looks like a single serving (a frozen pizza, a snack-sized bag of crisps or biscuits, or an individual bottle of drink), but the nutrition information on the packaging reveals that it's actually two or three servings. That means it's two or three times the calories, fat, sugar and everything else.

To save time at the supermarket, or to investigate a product without kids in tow, try reading about products online. Most food companies provide nutrition information and ingredient lists on their websites, making it easy to inform yourself before you hit the aisles.

3 Eat before you shop

When you're hungry, every pie, cake and bag of crisps is tantalizing. A full stomach will help you to ignore their overtures. If you have to head straight to the supermarket after work and don't have time to stop and eat before you go, buy a small, filling snack at the supermarket, such as a piece of fruit or a high-fibre bar, and eat it before you start shopping.

4 Hang out on the edge

The bulk of your trolley should be stacked with items from the outer aisles of the supermarket: fruit and veg, meats and dairy. Store layouts vary, but the fresh foods are almost always on the perimeter and the packaged goods in the

DECODING FOOD LABELS

Food labels provide lots of information that can help you achieve a healthy diet but are often confusing. Here's how to decipher them (you can also check out the Good Housekeeping Calorie Counter for additional advice).

Begin with reading the list of ingredients

The ingredients are listed in descending order of weight i.e. the most to the least. If an ingredient is mentioned in the name of a food, such as in 'apple pie', or is shown on the label, the amount of that ingredient contained in the food must be given as a percentage.

Read the nutrition label

The nutrients below must be listed per 100g (3½oz) or per 100ml (3½fl oz):

- Energy (kcal)
- Fat (g)
- Protein (g)
- Carbohydrate (g)

Should they want to, food manufacturers can include more nutritional information. If, however, a food product makes a health claim for a specific nutrient, the nutritional information for that nutrient must be listed; for example, if a food is described as low in salt, the salt content must be listed within the nutritional information.

Read the 'Traffic Light' or Guideline Daily Amount (GDA) labelling

'Traffic Light' labels are the labelling system approved by the Food Standards Agency, and tell you whether a packaged food has high, medium or low amounts of each of the nutrients in 100g (3½oz) of the food:

Green is used to show that a food is low in a nutrient.
Amber signals that a product contains medium levels of a nutrient.
Red represents high amounts and warns shoppers not to consume too much.

Many of the foods with traffic light colours will have a mixture of red, amber and green. The idea is that when you're choosing between similar products, you should go for more greens and ambers, and fewer reds.

Guideline Daily Amounts (GDAs) are a guide to how much energy and key nutrients the average healthy person needs in order to have a balanced diet. The GDAs for the most important nutrients listed on food labels are as follows:

GDAs		
	MEN	WOMEN
Fat (total)	95g (3¼oz)	65g (2½oz)
(of which saturates)	25g (1oz)	20g (¾oz)
Salt	6g (⅛oz)	6g (⅛oz)
Sugar *	120g (4oz)	90g (3¼oz)

* Total sugars includes sugars occurring naturally in foods as well as added sugars.

The labels show how much of a nutrient is in a portion of food; however, GDAs are a guide, not a target, and a maximum rather than a minimum. If you are a normal weight, you can aim to reach the GDA for calories, but you should try to eat no more than the GDAs for sugar, fat, saturates and salt.

Read the nutrition claims

Although these are defined by law, it's important to understand them alongside all the other information about a food; for example, a chocolate rice breakfast cereal could claim to be low in fat, but it could also be high in sugar and calories.

A general rule is to treat claims on food labels with caution. Something that claims to be low in fat may still contain the same number of calories as other similar versions or brands. The best way to decide whether a food is good enough for you is to look at the nutritional information and compare products.

Nutrition claims

Low-calorie	Contains fewer than 40 calories per 100g (3½oz)
Reduced-calorie	Contains at least 25 per cent fewer calories than the standard version
Low-fat	Contains less than 3g (⅛oz) of fat per 100g (3½oz) (for food) or 1.5g (¹⁄₁₆oz) of fat per 100ml (3½fl oz) (for liquids)
Reduced-fat	Contains 25 per cent less fat than a similar product
Less than 5 per cent fat	Contains less than 5g (⅛oz) of fat per 100g (3½oz) of the food
No added sugar	No sugar has been added as an ingredient. But the product may still contain high levels of natural sugars, such as in fruit juice or dried fruit
Low-sugar	Contains no more than 5g (⅛oz) sugar per 100g (3½oz)
Reduced-sugar	Contains 25 per cent less sugar than a similar product
Lite or light	No legal definition

If you (or your children) just can't seem to resist putting temptations into your trolley, try ordering your shopping online.

1 Use healthy search words

Try using search words such as 'low-fat', 'healthier' or 'light' when looking for foods such as sauces, ready meals, yogurts and desserts.

2 Make a list

Taking an hour to plan a week's meals will pay off, big time. To help, download the app Menu Planner (£1.99), which plans your meals, downloads your favourite recipes and tracks what you've got in your storecupboard.

3 Check the nutrition information

The majority of products provide detailed nutritional information on the pack. Check the calorie and nutritional value before you buy by clicking on the product image or name.

4 Use a supermarket comparison site

Try a grocery shopping site such as www. mysupermarket.com to ensure that you're getting the best deal – this can help you work out the cheapest place to shop and to see whether that special offer really is special.

5 Don't browse

The elimination of impulse buying may be online grocery shopping's biggest advantage, but there is still a temptation to browse fattening foods. Ignore or click past special offers that pop up before you reach the checkout.

Researchers in a multi-university study assigned 28 people to either a standard weight-loss programme or a one with online-ordered supermarket deliveries. After eight weeks, online buyers had fewer fattening products and less total food in their cupboards. Their secret? Virtual shopping trolleys make it easier to stick to a list and eliminate impulse shopping.

Check your local supermarkets for online shopping options, or try national services such as www.ocado.com, www.tesco.com, www.sainsburys.com, www.asda.com, or www.waitrose.com.

You'll not only save yourself from the consequences of diet-unfriendly impulse purchases but you'll also keep a little more cash in your pocket because you won't be blowing it on unnecessary extras.

Simple swaps

Swap this
228 calories for a 45g bag peanut M&Ms
For this
95 calories for 75g (3oz) grapes and 100g (3½oz) apple slices

It can be quite surprising how the simple choice of one cut of meat over another can save you calories – sometimes by substantial amount. Use our quick guide to see which cuts to choose for weight-loss results.

Good-for-your-waist foods

Gram for gram, beef tenderloin steaks contain about the same fat and calories as skinless chicken thighs. Chicken thighs are higher in fat and calories than breast meat, but if you remove the skin and excess fat, thighs fit into a good-for-you diet. They also provide 25 per cent more iron and over twice as much zinc as the same amount of breast meat. Pork tenderloin and boneless loin chops compare favourably, calorie-wise, with skinless chicken.

Stop the trolley for fatty fish!

Omega-3 fats are good for the heart, and can also be a boon to the waistline. In a multi-centre study involving 232 overweight volunteers on a reduced-calorie diet, researchers found that when the dieters ate a meal rich in fatty fish, they felt full for longer than those who had eaten a lean fish such as cod. The reason? High levels of omega-3s may prompt the body to produce more leptin – the hormone that signals fullness. This may lead you to eat less food throughout the day. One easy way to get these good-for-you fats is to use canned salmon, which is less expensive than fresh.

Stop the trolley for tofu!

Tofu's protein does the job of its meaty cousins. A Louisiana State University study found tofu to be a mighty diet food. Researchers tested it against chicken as an appetizer for 42 overweight women, and the participants who had tofu ate less food during the meal that followed. The secret: tofu seemed to quash hunger more than chicken.

DIET MADNESS	DIET MAKEOVER	YOU SAVE	SWAP TWICE A WEEK
Pork spare ribs *557 calories*	Pork tenderloin *271 calories*	*286 calories*	Drop 450g/0.5kg (1lb) in 6 weeks
Beef rib *441 calories*	Beef sirloin steak *291 calories*	*150 calories*	Drop 450g/0.5kg (1lb) in 11½ weeks
Mince *366 calories*	Lean mince *310 calories*	*56 calories*	Drop 450g/0.5kg (1lb) in 30 weeks
Chicken leg with skin *380 calories*	Chicken breast without skin *259 calories*	*121 calories*	Drop 450g/0.5kg (1lb) in 14 weeks

Note: weights per 175g (6oz) cooked meat, off the bone.

What do you do when you find yourself at home at lunchtime? Do you go for a quick sandwich? Yesterday's leftovers in the fridge? Or maybe you skip lunch completely and end up snacking all afternoon. Here are some midday ideas for when you're at home and trying to keep a check on your calories.

The fruits and vegetables on these pages are examples of some of the most nutrient-packed produce. Our picks are packed with vitamins, minerals and phytochemicals – health-boosting plant compounds – including lycopene (found in watermelon, grapefruit and tomatoes), lutein (in greens and broccoli), and carotenoids (in sweet potatoes, papaya and butternut squash).

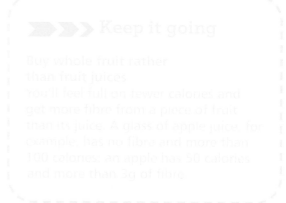

Fruit magic			
FRUIT SERVING	CALORIES	FIBRE	OTHER GOOD THINGS
½ grapefruit	24	1g	Pink varieties have more antioxidants and phytochemicals than their white or yellow cousins
1 kiwi fruit	29	1.1g	Gram for gram, kiwi fruits contain more vitamin C than an orange. They are also loaded with vitamin K, folate and potassium
½ mango	43	1.9g	Rich in vitamins A and C as well as a useful source of fibre, vitamin E and potassium
½ small punnet strawberries	34	1.4g	Packed with vitamin C, folate, fibre and flavour
1 slice of watermelon	62	0.2g	Has more lycopene than any other fruit or vegetable. Also rich in vitamins A and C

Buy pre-prepared produce

With already peeled, cut and washed fruit and vegetables to hand, you'll be less likely to turn to unhealthy choices. Although they cost more than whole produce, they're hassle-free and time-saving.

Pre-washed salad leaves It's easy to eat salads more often when all you have to do is open a bag and dress it. Look for dark leaves (such as baby spinach, rocket, corn salad and watercress), which pack more nutrition per bite than standard lettuce.

Prepared fruit If you're counting on fruit to help you through a sweet craving, it's got to be ready when the need strikes. Prepared fruit can also reduce the chance that you'll buy a whole fruit and forget it in your fridge.

Ready-made coleslaw Talk about versatility in a bag. Look for plain coleslaw (sans the fatty dressing, of course) and try it sautéed with a little oil for a quick side dish, mix it with vegetables for a stir-fry, or use it to bulk up home-made or canned soups.

Stop the trolley for spinach!

Spinach nutritionally outscores even the much-praised broccoli, with its long list of vitamins and minerals. This leafy wonder is also one of the richest sources of lutein, a plant chemical that protects against age-related blindness. It's convenient, too: just open a bag of pre-washed baby spinach for salads or sandwiches. Or pop it in the microwave for two to three minutes for a convenient side dish. To economize, cook a bag of frozen spinach, which is just as nutritious.

Vegetable magic

VEGETABLE SERVING	CALORIES	FIBRE	OTHER GOOD THINGS
3 broccoli florets	26	2.1g	Rich in vitamins K and C, carotenoids, calcium, iron and potassium
8 Brussels sprouts	34	3.3g	Contains vitamins K and C, carotenoids, calcium, iron and potassium
2 handfuls salad leaves such as baby spinach or watercress	20	1.7g	Rich in vitamins A, C and K, as well as folate, potassium, magnesium, iron, lutein and other phytochemicals
¼ butternut squash	29	1.3g	Loaded with potassium, magnesium, and vitamins A and C
1 medium sweet potato	150	4.3g	Packed with carotenoids, vitamin C, potassium and fibre

Wholegrain foods can help you Drop a Dress Size because they contain more fibre and are more filling, which leaves you feeling satisfied. As a bonus, they have more healthy nutrients than refined grain-based foods. To get the most nutrients per serving, look for products that are 100 per cent whole grain.

IT'S A WHOLE GRAIN IF IT'S CALLED:	IT'S NOT A WHOLE GRAIN IF IT'S CALLED:
Wholegrain or brown rice	Cornflour
Buckwheat	Cornmeal
Bulgur or cracked wheat	Basmati rice
Millet	Enriched flour
Quinoa	White long-grain rice or short-grain rice
Sorghum	Rice flour
Triticale	Rye flour
Wheat berries	Stone-ground wheat (if wholegrain, label should say 'stone-ground wholemeal')
Wholegrain barley or pearl barley	Unbleached wheat flour
Corn	Maize flour
Oats or oatmeal	Wheat flour
Jumbo oats	
Wholegrain rye flour	
Spelt	
Wholemeal/wholewheat	

Ready-to-eat food isn't always an unhealthy option. Check out these top five convenience grain dishes, which won't break your Drop a Dress Size plan.

Get the wholegrain truth

If the label on a convenience food dish does not state '100 per cent whole grain', check the ingredients list for refined-grain culprits.

Choosing pasta

Opt for 100 per cent wholegrain pasta rather than white pasta. Bear in mind that some wholegrain pastas are chewier than others and some shapes taste better than others. There are plenty to choose from, so if at first you don't succeed, try (another brand) and try (another shape – say, linguine, if you didn't like the spaghetti) again. Or choose buckwheat, millet or corn pasta.

1 Uncle Ben's express wholegrain rice

Ready-cooked wholegrain rice in a pouch that you just heat up in the microwave:
201 calories per ½ pouch, 125g (4oz)

2 Tilda steamed wholegrain pilau

A blend of cumin, curry leaf and fenugreek infuses this delicious, ready-cooked wholegrain basmati pilau with flavour:
164 calories per ½ pouch, 125g (4oz)

3 Merchant Gourmet ready-to-eat wholesome mixed grains

The goodness of bulgur wheat, quinoa, lentils and soya flakes in olive oil, which you simply heat in the microwave:
254 calories per ½ pouch, 125g (4oz)

4 Food Doctor wholesome pot of bulgur wheat and quinoa

A handy snack pot of savoury bulgur wheat and quinoa with asparagus, leek and mint:
254 calories per pot, 65g (2½oz)

5 Food Doctor easy grain organic cereal, pulses and beans

A nutrient-dense mixture of quinoa, lentils, spelt and kidney beans, ready to eat or to heat:
297 calories per pouch, 225g (8oz)

Milk, yogurt, eggs and cheese are all great sources of calcium and protein. In fact, see The Calcium Connection opposite to learn how eating more calcium-rich dairy foods may help you to lose weight.

Five healthy cheeses

Cathedral City lighter Cheddar
78 calories per 25g (1oz) serving

Philadelphia Extra Light mini-tubs
38 calories per 35g tub

The Laughing Cow light cheese portion
25 calories per 17.5g portion

Leerdammer Lightlife slices
55 calories per slice, 20g (¾oz)

Mini Babybel light
42 calories per piece

Five healthy yogurts

Danone Activia fat-free yogurt (any flavour)
65 calories per 125g pot

Fage Total 0% yogurt (natural)
97 calories per 175g pot

Yeo Valley organic probiotic yogurt (any flavour)
123 calories per 120g pot

Danone Shape Delights mango and peach 0% yogurt
72 calories per 120g pot

Müller Light cherry yogurt
82 calories per 175g pot

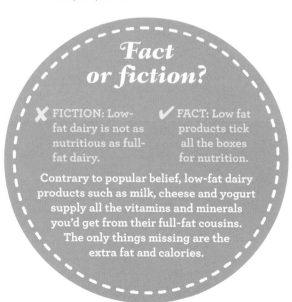

Fact or fiction?

✗ FICTION: Low-fat dairy is not as nutritious as full-fat dairy.

✓ FACT: Low fat products tick all the boxes for nutrition.

Contrary to popular belief, low-fat dairy products such as milk, cheese and yogurt supply all the vitamins and minerals you'd get from their full-fat cousins. The only things missing are the extra fat and calories.

The skinny on yogurt

Look for yogurt with no more than 125 calories and 2g of saturated fat per serving.

The low-down on cheese

Look for cheese with no more than 70 calories and 3g of saturated fat per 25g (1oz) serving (including hard cheese, soft cheese, cheese spreads, and goat's cheese). Cottage cheese and ricotta cheese should have no more than 100 calories and 2g of saturated fat per serving.

The calcium connection

Eating more calcium-rich dairy foods may help you to Drop a Dress Size. Studies have found that adults who eat a calcium-rich, high-dairy diet lose more weight and fat than those who consume a low-dairy diet with the same number of calories. Researchers speculate that calcium-rich dairy foods may boost the body's fat-burning ability after a meal.

Stop the trolley for eggs!

When researchers tracked people on a low-cal diet, they found that those who ate two eggs for breakfast lost 65 per cent more weight than those who had a bagel – even though they consumed the same number of calories. (Plus, the egg eaters' cholesterol levels didn't go up.) They shed the extra pounds because they felt full after breakfast and ate fewer calories throughout the day.

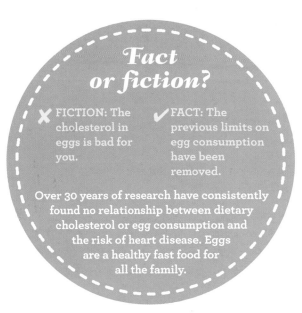

Fact or fiction?

✘ FICTION: The cholesterol in eggs is bad for you.

✔ FACT: The previous limits on egg consumption have been removed.

Over 30 years of research have consistently found no relationship between dietary cholesterol or egg consumption and the risk of heart disease. Eggs are a healthy fast food for all the family.

Are you afraid that the temptations of the ready-meal food aisles will derail your Drop a Dress Size efforts? Here are our guidelines for ready meals, pizzas, ice cream and more.

Look for ready meals and pizzas and with no more than 400 calories and 12g of fat, and at least 3g of fibre per meal or 175g (6oz) portion of pizza (about a third of a 25.5cm (10in) pizza). Opt for wholegrain choices whenever you can find them. Round out your meal with vegetables or a salad – they take little time to prepare but will provide that all-important balance as well as filling you up.

Svelte ready meals
A pick of the best ready meals:

Tesco Light Choices chicken breast with tikka masala sauce
190 calories per pack

The City Kitchen skinny Mediterranean orzo prawns
320 calories per pack

Sainsbury's Be Good To Yourself tomato and basil chicken
373 calories per pack

Asda Good For You beef bourguignon
325 calories per pack

Innocent moussaka veg pot
288 calories per pot

Waitrose LoveLife You Count cottage pie
338 calories per pack

Stewed! One-Pot Meals Thai green chicken and noodles
351 calories per pot

Choice pizzas

Pizzas you can enjoy:

Waitrose 12-inch hand-stretched, thin and crispy fire-roasted pepper and courgette pizza
370 calories per 1/3 pizza

Pizza Express 8-inch Light vitabella pizza
215 calories per 1/2 pizza

Tesco thin-crust mighty vegetable pizza
325 calories per 1/2 pizza

Sainsbury's thin and crispy supreme 10-inch pizza
400 calories per 1/2 pizza

Asda ultra-thin marinated chicken and garlic spinach pizza
297 calories per pizza

Weight Watchers chicken arrabiata pizza oval
223 calories per pizza

Dessert treats

Desserts for occasional indulgence:

Carte d'Or Light vanilla ice cream
140 calories per 100ml (3½fl oz)

Yog Fat-free Wonderful pomegranate frozen yogurt
85 calories per 100ml (3½fl oz)

Ben & Jerry's chocolate fudge brownie frozen yogurt
150 calories per 100ml (3½fl oz)

Saintly snacks to kill your cravings

You're craving ... chocolate
Swap this
260 calories for a 49g bar of Dairy Milk
For this
40 calories for an Options Belgian hot chocolate drink

You're craving ... ice cream
Swap this
675 calories for ½ tub, 250ml (9fl oz), Ben & Jerry's cookie dough ice cream
For this
93 calories per 100ml (3½fl oz) stick Skinny Cow caramel shortbread ice cream

You're craving ... something salty and crunchy
Swap this
500 calories per ½ tube, 95g (3½oz), Pringles
For this
75 calories per 24g bag Ryvita minis

1 Skinny Cow mint double choc stick
94 calories per stick

150ml pot Yoo Moo strawbmoo frozen yogurt
134 calories per carton

On the go and no time for exercise? These clever toning moves use all your major muscles and are great for burning calories.

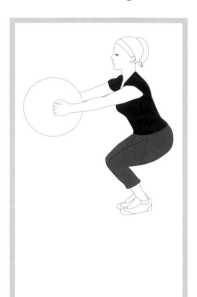

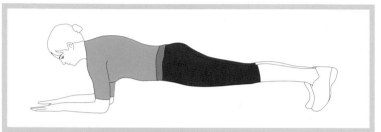

Plank
Lie face down with your hands either side of your head and your elbows on the ground. Push yourself up, keeping your weight on your forearms and feet. Your elbows should be bent at 90°. Keep your back straight. Hold this position for 15–30 seconds.

Squat and arm raise
Hold a ball or weight in front of you and squat down, keeping your back nice and straight. As you push back up, raise your arms straight up above your head. Return to the starting position and repeat 10–12 times.

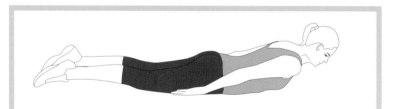

Back extension
Lie face down on the floor, arms by your sides. Lift your head and shoulders off the floor, still facing the ground. Hold this position for a few seconds and then lower yourself back down. Repeat 6–8 times.

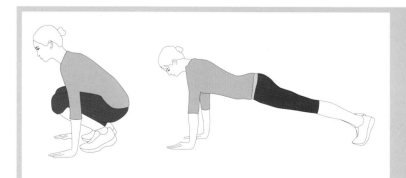

Squat thrusts
From a standing position, crouch down to squat with your hands on the floor, shoulder-width apart, near your feet. Now jump back with your feet so that you're in a press-up position. Jump forward to your original squat position with your hands still on the floor. Repeat 10 times.

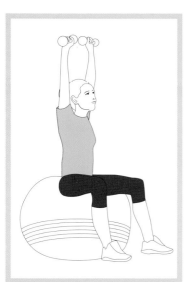

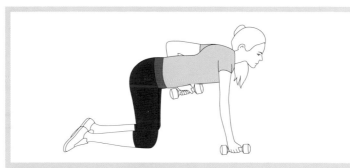

Kneeling row
Kneeling on all fours, hold a weight in your left hand and support your body weight on your right hand. Pull the weight up towards your armpit. Hold for a second before lowering the weight. Keep your back still and straight. Repeat 10–12 times.

Seated press
Sit on a chair or a stability/Swiss ball. Hold a pair of dumb-bells, hands facing forwards, level with your shoulders. Press the dumb-bells upwards and inwards until they almost touch over your head. Straighten your arms but do not lock your elbows. Hold for a count of one. Lower the dumb-bells slowly to the starting position and repeat 10–15 times.

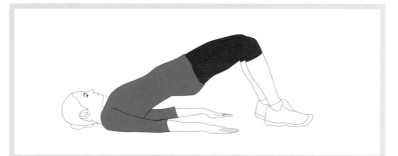

Bridge
Lie on your back with your legs bent and feet flat on the floor. Lift your hips off the floor until you form a straight line between knees, hips and shoulders. Lower your hips back down to the floor. Repeat 10–12 times.

Half push-ups
Lie face down on the floor with your hands next to your shoulders on the floor. Keeping your knees on the floor and your ankles crossed, slowly push yourself up until your arms are straight, then lower yourself back down so that your arms are bent at 90° and your nose almost touches the floor. Repeat 10–12 times.

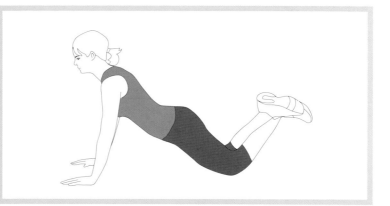

FAT-BUSTING WEEKDAY MEAL PLANNER

	MONDAY	TUESDAY	WEDNESDAY	THURSDAY	FRIDAY
BREAKFAST (about 350 calories)	40g (1½oz) Kellogg's Just Right, 75g (3oz) berries, 1 tbsp chopped nuts, 125ml (4fl oz) skimmed milk	1 toasted wholemeal muffin spread with a little butter and 2 tsp jam; 1 orange	Porridge made with 40g (1½oz) oats, 250ml (9fl oz) skimmed milk; 1 banana	2 slices of wholemeal toast spread with a little butter and 1 tbsp honey	1 boiled egg and 1 slice of wholemeal toast with a little butter; ½ grapefruit
LUNCH (about 500 calories)	Wholemeal tuna sandwich (2 slices of wholemeal bread, 75g/3oz canned tuna, mustard); side salad with 1 tbsp olive oil; 1 apple	Summer Couscous (p. 136); ½ small punnet strawberries	1 wholemeal pitta filled with 2 tbsp hummus and lots of salad leaves; 1 apple and 1 x 125ml pot low-fat yogurt	Tuna Salad (p. 137) with 1 wholemeal roll and a little butter; 1 pear	2 slices of wholemeal toast with 200g (7oz) baked beans; a leafy salad with 1 tbsp oil dressing; 2 plums
DINNER (about 500 calories)	150g (5oz) steak fillet, 175g (6oz) new potatoes, green beans and carrots; 100ml (3½fl oz) Carte d'Or Light vanilla ice cream	115g grilled salmon, 150g (5oz) grilled courgettes/ aubergines/ peppers, 3 tbsp cooked wholegrain rice; 150g (5oz) blueberries	Pork and Noodle Stir-fry (p. 140)	Tomato and Butter Bean Stew (p. 134), 3 tbsp wholegrain rice; 150g (5oz) fruit salad	Sardines with Mediterranean Vegetables (p. 131); 125g (4oz) new potatoes
SNACK (about 100 calories)	1 Skinny Cow mint double choc stick	20g (¾oz) almonds	1 banana	1 x 100ml (3½fl oz) Yog fat-free Wonderful pomegranate frozen yogurt	1 Laughing Cow Light cheese portion plus 3 Ryvita wholegrain crispbreads

The largest, longest-running study of successful dieters, the National Weight Control Registry in the US, tracked the progress of more than 5,000 people who lost an average of 30kg (4 stone 10lb) and kept it off for five and a half years. So how did they do it? They shifted their mindset and developed healthy habits. Try it for yourself:

• Get organized. Researchers found that it was the people who were structured and disciplined in their approach to life who were the most successful at keeping weight off – the 'maintainers'.

• Keep moving. Ninety per cent of successful maintainers exercise (gently) for an hour or more a day – the equivalent of a four-mile daily walk.

• Weigh yourself every day. Cut back on what you eat if your weight goes up more than 900g (2lb). Research shows that people who abandon regular weight checks are more likely to overeat.

• Eat breakfast every day and never skip meals. This strategy will stop hunger pangs and overeating.

• Spend no more than ten hours a week watching TV. Studies show that people who eat while doing other things, like watching TV or working on a computer, consistently underestimate how much they've eaten.

• Be consistent. Successful maintainers don't skip meals or 'cheat' at weekends.

• Don't lapse during Christmas and holidays. Maintainers pay even more attention to what they eat at 'food overload' times, take regular exercise and check their weight.

• Stick to a low-fat, low-calorie diet. The good news is that the longer you do it, the easier it gets. People who managed to maintain their weight for two to five years were far more likely to keep it off for good.

Fitness first

Regular physical activity prevents illness, boosts your mood, relieves stress and helps you Drop a Dress Size faster.

If you're confused about how much exercise you need to do in order to lose weight, you're not alone. Is it 20 minutes a day – or 30? Or 45? Does it have to be done all at once, or can it be broken up? Should it be aerobic exercise or strength training, and do you need to do a high-intensity workout every time?

Losing weight boils down to a very simple equation: calories in versus calories out. It's not about gimmicks, fads, or tricks – just basic arithmetic. If you burn more calories than you eat, you will lose weight. So follow the Drop a Dress Size eating advice, add exercise, and you'll see faster results. Remember, a deficit of 3,500 calories, either because you eat fewer calories or because you burn more calories by working out – or both – will result in a 450g/0.5kg (1lb) weight loss.

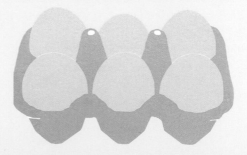

1 Follow the pleasure principle

What do ice skating, hula-hooping, Zumba (Latin-rhythm aerobic dancing), kickboxing and swimming have in common? They're all fun – and they all burn calories while you're doing them. Research shows that when you're enjoying yourself, you're more likely to stick with an activity. And the more you stick with it, the more pounds you'll drop.

2 Exercise family-style

Choose activities you can do as a family, like a bike ride, playing frisbee or bowling, to keep everyone healthy. Find an interesting short walk around a local country park or the grounds of a stately home. Or, more simply, kick around a football, go ice-skating, or take your dog on a really long walk once or twice a week on top of normal dog-walking duties.

Even if you are not the outdoorsy type, exercise can still be fun for the whole family. With Nintendo's Wii Fit game, even the most committed couch potatoes will enjoy standing on the Wii Balance Board and following on-screen instructions for yoga, aerobics, strength training – and even walking a tightrope and hula-hooping! You earn points for good performance and get feedback on how you can improve.

3 Learn a new skill

Always wanted to try in-line skating, golf, cross-country skiing or ballroom dancing? Would you like to join a running club or take up yoga, tennis or salsa dancing? Do it! You'll learn something new and Drop a Dress Size at the same time. Check local organizations or your local sports centre for affordable classes. For even more fun, gather a group of friends to learn a new, calorie-burning activity together.

4 Break it up

If you don't have a full hour (or even 30 minutes) to dedicate to exercise each day, try doing several mini-workouts throughout the day. Two 15-minute workouts are just as effective as a single one of 30 minutes, and a great way to prevent boredom.

Dividing up your workout can even help you stay more dedicated to losing weight. Researchers at the University of Pittsburgh found that people who exercised for ten minutes, several times a day, were able to exercise an average of 35 minutes longer per week than subjects who were told to do the same amount of exercise in just one session each day. (Consider that the average person who exercises does only 60 to 90 minutes per week. An additional 35 minutes on top of that is an increase of roughly 33–55 per cent!) They also burned more calories and improved their cardio-respiratory health.

5 Go at a reasonable pace

Suppose you haven't exercised in a while. After a sudden urge to get fit and lose weight, should you immediately go for a 60-minute run or lift 6.8kg (15lb) dumb-bells at the gym? Of course not! Doing this will only risk injury. Even if you avoid hurting yourself, you'll be convinced that exercise is too difficult and then quit before you've really started. The solution? Start slowly and work at an intensity that feels comfortable. Begin with a 15-minute leisurely walk, and then, when you feel ready, try the Drop a Dress Size fat-blasting walking plan (see pages 98–101). Branch out and try new activities such as water aerobics, t'ai chi or bike riding. The best part: the entire time your body is adapting to increased exercise, you're burning calories and on your way to dropping the weight.

10 REASONS TO BE ACTIVE

If you've always been inclined to avoid over-exerting yourself, you may be surprised to learn how great you can feel after relatively little exercise. It's easy to get the activity bug – once you start to feel the benefit, you'll soon be building up your exercise quota and getting great results. Here's why exercise is so good for you:

1 It burns fat
Regular activity burns fat, helping you lose weight faster and preventing further weight gain.

2 It benefits your health
Regular activity halves your risk of developing heart disease, reduces the risk of having a stroke, helps lower blood pressure and reduces the chance of developing diabetes.

3 It strengthens your muscles
Doing strength or toning exercises three times a week will prevent the age-related loss of 2.3–3.2kg (5–7lb) muscle per decade that happens after the age of about 30.

4 It makes your heart stronger
Activity strengthens your heart muscle, allowing it to pump blood efficiently around your body with each heartbeat.

5 It relieves stiffness
Stretching exercises relieve stiffness, improve your range of movement and increase your flexibility.

6 It's good for your bones
By undertaking weight-bearing exercise such as walking, running and dancing, you can slow bone loss, which can lead to osteoporosis (thinning of the bones).

7 It improves mood and reduces stress
Regular activity can reduce stress, anxiety and depression – you'll relax more easily and feel better about yourself.

8 It gives you a good posture
All activities improve your posture, balance, strength, suppleness and mobility.

9 It enhances your self-esteem
Regular exercise improves your self-image, so you'll have a greater desire to eat healthily too.

10 It gives you more energy
You'll be able to cope better with your daily routine and have energy to spare.

 Step on it!

Targets
Think big, but set yourself small, manageable targets week by week. You need to visualize your end goal, but take small steps to get there and mark your successes along the way.

You already have the best fat-burning equipment: your feet. The secret is knowing how to use them. Our Drop a Dress Size fat-blasting walking programme will help you find the right pace for you – whether that's an easy stroll or a heart-pumping workout. Counting those steps with a pedometer will help to ensure that you melt off the pounds.

The Drop a Dress Size fat-blasting walking plan

Going for a walk may be as easy as putting on your trainers and stepping outside, but if you want to Drop a Dress Size fast, it's best to have a plan. Our programme is specifically designed to bump your body into a higher calorie- and fat-burning zone, so you'll lose weight and firm up. Combine this walking plan with the calorie cutbacks, and you could Drop a Dress Size in about two and a half weeks!

You'll do four 30-minute walking workouts a week – ideally on Tuesday, Thursday, Saturday and Sunday. The step-by-step details are charted out for you on page 100, but here's a quick breakdown of your activities for each day – and how they'll make a difference to your weight loss.

Tuesdays Walk normally … then speed up for one to two minutes. Go as fast as your feet will carry you, but try to maintain good form (see Keep it Going, opposite). This extra 'fast lane' push makes your metabolism work overtime so that you burn more calories post-exercise.

Thursdays March up inclines. If there are hills nearby, try to include some gentle ones in your walk. Walking on an incline forces your muscles and cardiovascular system to work harder and burns one-third more calories than walking on the flat. It works just as well on the way down, as downhill walking tones your bottom and thighs, too. On treadmills, simply increase the incline to about 4 per cent. No hills? No

treadmill? Get the same muscle boost by walking up one or more flights of stairs for 60 seconds. You'll see results fast: Tufts University researchers reported that older adults who added lean muscle tissue through resistance exercises three days a week for 12 weeks, boosted their resting metabolism by about 7 per cent.

Saturdays Take a brisk walk to build stamina and strength. Find a pace that's quick enough for you to feel a burn, but not so tough that you can't sustain it for at least 20 minutes.

Sundays This is your day of rest. Translation: you can walk as slowly or as fast as you like. Just make sure you get outdoors and hit the pavement.

Find your pace

The workout is divided into four pace levels: easy, moderate, challenging and hard. What's easy for one person can be hard for another – you may feel pooped after a brisk walk, whereas a friend might only feel like that after a near-jog. How should you work out your best-results speed? Talk as you're walking, and gauge how hard it is for you to speak, then see where you score on the guide below.

Easy The pace of your walk is so effortless that you can chat freely (no panting, no breathlessness).

Moderate You can still chat, but you need to pause occasionally to catch your breath.

Challenging You have little breath for small talk, but you can still manage to talk in short sentences.

Hard You can get out a 'yes', 'no' or 'perhaps' – but you really can't talk right now!

SPEED UP YOUR STRIDE

Moderate exercise provides proven heart benefits, but you may have to speed up the pace to earn them. Studies have shown that, left to their own estimates of what's fast enough, many people aren't getting the fitness boost they think they are. To find the best speed, researchers from San Diego State University measured energy output as 97 people walked on a treadmill, then translated the participants' speeds to a formula that everyone can use. The right pace? About 100 steps a minute. To load your iPod with songs that set the tempo, go to www.DjBPMStudio.com, click on 'Index by BPM' (that's beats per minute), then choose 100. Check your pace with a pedometer. Or see Listen to Lose on page 105 for our top five exercise songs.

Did you know?

The average woman will burn about 300 calories an hour when walking. If you walk for 30 minutes, six days a week, you'll lose about a pound a week, without eating less – that's almost 6.3kg (1 stone) a year.

 ### Step on it!

Find a new walk
Variety will keep you motivated. Don't just stick with one route – have several and alternate between them. To find new places to walk, check out Walking for Health's walk finder at www.whi.org.uk/walkfinder.

WALKING PLAN

Four 30-minute walks a week will help you Drop a Dress Size. Follow the four-week programme below. See page 99 for an explanation of the pace levels.

WEEK 1	
TUESDAY	**SATURDAY**
Warm up for 5 minutes at EASY level	Warm up for 5 minutes at EASY level
Increase to HARD for 1 minute, then reduce pace to MODERATE for 1 minute. Repeat five times	Increase to MODERATE for 5 minutes
Finish the last 15 minutes at MODERATE	Pick up the pace to CHALLENGING for 5 minutes
THURSDAY	**SUNDAY**
Warm up for 5 minutes at EASY level	Walk as slowly or as quickly as you like for 30 minutes
Increase to MODERATE for 10 minutes	Don't forget to warm up and cool down
Walk at CHALLENGING for 1–2 minutes (uphill, at 4 per cent incline, or up the stairs), then cool down by walking on a flat surface for 1–2 minutes. Repeat once	
Finish the last 7–11 minutes at MODERATE	
WEEKS 2–4: REPEAT	

TO LOSE MORE, WALK THE RIGHT WAY
For a workout that's more than just leg exercise, copy this fitness instructor's total-body style:
• Walk tall with your chin parallel to the ground, eyes focused ahead – don't look down.
• Hold your arms at a 90° angle and pump them forward and backwards, with your hands in loose fists. Stand upright, with your shoulders back and relaxed.
• Always place your heel down first and let the middle of your foot and toes follow.

Here are a few things to consider before you decide where to go for your walk.

INDOORS (treadmill)	OUTDOORS (pavement, track, footpath or road)
No ice, sleet, rain, snow, or darkness to worry about	The sun in the sky, the wind in your hair, fresh air
A crèche in a gym or a sleeping baby at home means you can squeeze in a workout when convenient	You can bring the kids along; little ones can ride in carriers or all-terrain pushchairs
Consistency, smooth surface; there's no stumbling on tree roots or cracked pavements	Walking on an imperfect surface will burn slightly more calories (1–5 per cent)
If you're visiting an unfamiliar area, you can play it safe and go to the hotel fitness centre	An excellent way to explore a new city – get a guidebook and take a walking tour
Offers a super-controlled workout; you can precisely adjust the speed and incline	Great variety of terrain; trekking up a hill can increase calorie-burn, and since there is no way to flatten the incline, you're forced to push yourself

Count your steps

Here's the thing about steps: they add up, and pedometers offer a lot of motivation. A Stanford University review study confirmed it: people who wear a pedometer take more than 2,000 extra steps a day – that's about a mile!

An inactive individual takes, on average, between 1,000 and 3,000 steps per day. If you take 5,000 additional steps each day, you could burn about 200 extra calories (this is an estimate – your weight and the speed you walk at both factor in). Up it to 10,000 total steps at the weekend, and you'll burn that much more. So, strap on a pedometer (pick one based on durability, accuracy, performance and ease of use) and start stepping!

Take longish strolls with your spouse, children or friends. Walk the dog around the block a few extra times. Use the stairs instead of the escalator. Walk to your local shops, church, post office or wherever. Walk every day, as much as you can.

Investing in a pair of trainers will help you to tone up and encourage you to exercise more. Here's how to choose the right ones:

1 Know your feet

Do the wet footprint test. Make footprints on a tiled floor with damp feet. If the print shows almost the whole of the sole of your foot, you probably have a low arch. With a regular arch, the band between the heel and forefoot will be about half the width of the foot, and with a high arch you'll see only a narrow band between the forefoot and arch. Take this into consideration when buying trainers.

2 Buy from a reputable sports shop

A good sports shop will employ properly trained staff. If you are on a budget, you should never have to pay more than £60 for a good pair of trainers. If you use them once or twice a week, they should last you about a year.

3 Find the right shoes

If you have a low arch, you need a stability trainer with extra support on the inside to prevent your feet rolling inwards. If you have a high arch, go for a pair of cushioned trainers. If you have a regular arch, choose neutral trainers.

4 Get the right fit

You will probably need a half-size larger for trainers than for your regular shoes. There should be a thumb's width at the end of the shoe. This will allow for the swelling of your feet and movement within the shoe, which takes place as you walk or run.

5 Take it easy

Don't do a five-mile walk in a new pair of shoes – break them in gently by wearing them around the house or garden.

Perfect posture

An improved posture could be your shortcut to a leaner, slimmer shape. Try these simple exercises.

Don't slouch Stand or sit up straight, and push your shoulder blades together and down. Increasing the width between your shoulders can make your waist look thinner and reduces the risk of neck and shoulder pain.

Stand tall Stand evenly on two feet, with your back straight, knees soft and buttocks squeezed. Imagine a string in the middle of your head pulling you up. Lengthening your spine instantly adds a few inches, making you look longer and fitter. It also reduces tummy bulge and lower back strain.

Strengthen your core These deep muscles around your back and pelvis stabilize and strengthen your body. Lie on your back, knees bent, feet flat, spine in neutral and your legs hip-distance apart. Pull in your lower abdomen as far as you can, as if you were zipping up a tight pair of jeans. Hold for a count of ten, breathe normally and repeat 10 times.

 Step on it!

Get the gear
Wear cushioned, supportive trainers that allow you to wiggle your toes inside. Also, wear layers of loose, comfortable clothing that you can layer up or peel off as needed.

If you want to get in shape but you're not up for a marathon, try some of these less taxing alternatives.

Pilates

Named after Joseph Pilates (pronounced 'puh-lah-tees'), who developed a set of floor exercises 70 years ago, this workout combines strength, flexibility, balance, core-strengthening and control training with resistance exercises. It's done individually or in groups, with or without specific pieces of specially designed equipment. A workout lasts 45 minutes–1½ hours, and although it's not aerobic at lower levels, advanced students can get cardiovascular benefit.

You burn 168 calories per 1-hour session.

Water workouts

Exercising in water is increasingly popular with people who have been injured by high-impact workouts. Participants can walk on underwater treadmills or perform arm, leg and abdominal exercises. Minute for minute, it burns fewer calories than the same exercises performed on land, but many people find they can train for longer, in part because the water pressure helps the blood circulate so that the heart doesn't have to work as hard.

You burn 270 calories per 1-hour session.

T'ai chi

This ancient Chinese practice improves strength, flexibility, concentration and balance by combining mental discipline with physical movement. When done correctly, t'ai chi can raise your heart rate to 60 per cent of maximum, qualifying as moderate exercise. The thighs and hips do much of the work, just as in high-impact aerobics – but without the jumping. And it just may keep you young: aerobic capacity, a measure of how the heart, lungs and circulatory system are working,

declines with age, but one study demonstrated that t'ai chi practitioners managed to slow the process through regular practice.

You burn 270 calories per 1-hour session.

Yoga

Now practised by more than 2 million Brits, yoga improves flexibility, muscle strength and endurance. It consists of deep-breathing exercises and postures or poses. Yoga also involves muscle toning and some aerobic movement. The poses can be adapted to any fitness level. As you increase the depth of practice, the benefits increase. It's best to start with a supervised class, so that you learn how to do the positions correctly, otherwise you risk injury and may not get the full effect.

You burn 200 calories per 1-hour session.

Ballet

You don't have to be a little girl with dreams of becoming a prima ballerina to enjoy this graceful, exacting form of dance, which is becoming a popular way for adults to stretch and strengthen underused muscles and to improve balance, flexibility and coordination. An added benefit is improved posture: ballet moves teach you to align your body and they also promote discipline in a fitness regime.

You burn 320 calories per 1-hour session.

All calorie burn-off calculations are based on a 63kg (10 stone) woman.

EASY WAYS TO BURN 100 CALORIES

Ready to Drop a Dress Size faster? Decide how much time you have, then choose any one of these activities.*

10 MINUTES	Run around the block Skip with a rope quickly Work out to a step aerobics video
15 MINUTES	Climb up and down your stairs at a moderate pace Play touch football with the family Swim laps, any style, at a leisurely pace Go roller-skating Hit some tennis balls
20 MINUTES	Power-walk (walking at a brisk pace while pumping the arms) Weed the garden Turn up the music and dance around the room
25 MINUTES	Rake the lawn and bag the leaves Cycle at a leisurely speed Go horse riding Vacuum Wash the floors Play a serious table tennis match
30 MINUTES	Throw a frisbee around Go ballroom dancing Lift light weights Wash your car Sweep the floors
35 MINUTES	Dust the house Practise the piano or violin Set the table and prepare a meal Play catch with your kids Clear the table and do the washing up
40 MINUTES	Iron your clothes Window shop Unload the dryer and fold the laundry Go shopping at the supermarket

Fact or fiction?

✘ FICTION: Your body won't burn fat unless you exercise for more than 20 minutes.

✔ FACT: You burn fat around the clock, whether you're exercising or not.

For the biggest calorie-burn, exercise as hard as you comfortably can (you should still be able to carry on a conversation) for as long as you can.

* Calorie burn-off calculations based on a 63kg (10 stone) woman.

TOP 5 EASY WAYS TO BURN MORE CALORIES

1 Speed up

Raise your walking tempo from a leisurely 2 mph to a brisk 3½ mph and you'll increase your calorie-burn by more than a third.

2 Stand up

Standing up uses 50 per cent more calories than sitting. Pace around and you'll burn even more.

3 Fidget

US researchers found that one reason why some people stay slim is because of non-exercise activity thermogenesis (NEAT): the calories burned doing unstructured activities such as taking the stairs, popping down the corridor to the office water cooler, bustling about with chores at home – or simply fidgeting.

4 Eat small, frequent meals

Each time you eat, your body uses calories to digest the food.

5 Pump your arms when you walk

If you also take the hilly route, you'll increase your calorie-burn even more.

LISTEN TO LOSE

People who work out to music could lose twice as much as those who exercise in silence, suggests recent research, because music helps you stick to your workout for longer. Make your next exercise session really sing with our exercise song picks. (We've included the beats per minute, because experts recommend walking at a rate of at least 100 steps per minute to maximize benefits.)
- 'Bad Romance' (119 bpm), Lady Gaga
- 'Tik Tok' (120 bpm), Ke$ha
- 'Teenage Dream' (120 bpm), Katy Perry
- 'Single Ladies' (197 bpm), Beyoncé
- 'Don't Stop the Music' (123 bpm), Rihanna

 STEP ON IT!

Laugh more often
A study from Vanderbilt University showed that you can burn up to 40 calories by laughing, genuinely, for 10–15 minutes.

This beginner's walk/jog programme allows you to build from nothing to running for almost 20 minutes within four weeks. You can do the workout outside or on a treadmill at the gym. Allow at least a day between workouts when you begin.

	DAY 1	DAY 2	DAY 3	DAY 4	DAY 5	DAY 6	DAY 7
WEEK 1	Walk 3 mins, run 1 min. (× 4)	Rest	Walk 2 mins, run 1 min. (× 5)	Rest	Walk 1 min., run 1 min. (× 7)	Rest	Rest or walk for 30 mins
WEEK 2	Walk 2 mins, run 2 mins (× 4)	Rest	Walk 2 mins, run 2 mins (× 5)	Rest	Walk 2 mins, run 3 mins (× 4)	Rest	Rest or walk for 30 mins
WEEK 3	Walk 2 mins, run 3 mins (× 5)	Rest	Walk 2 mins, run 2 mins (× 6)	Rest	Walk 2 mins, run 4 mins (× 3)	Rest	Rest or walk for 30 mins
WEEK 4	Walk 2 mins, run 5 mins (× 3)	Rest	Walk 1 min., run 3 mins (× 6)	Rest	Jog for 15–20 mins without stopping (walk if needed)	Rest	Rest or walk for 30 mins

 Step on it!

Find a walking pal
There will be days when you don't feel like walking but a walking pal does, and vice versa, so you'll motivate each other to keep going. For a local buddy, try www.go4awalk.com.

1 Sleep more, weigh less

Exercising won't work if you're not going to bed early enough. A study in the *Annals of Internal Medicine* found that people who slept just 5½ hours per night lost 55 per cent less fat than those who slept for 8½ hours. What they did shed, sadly, was muscle.

2 Tone up

Walking helps to tone you up. Researchers found that walking 30 minutes a day helped people to lose body fat, and it trimmed their waist size and built muscle.

3 Just keep moving

Although the Department of Health recommends 150 minutes of exercise per week for weight management, the truth is, when you are trying to Drop a Dress Size, doing any exercise for any length of time, at any intensity, will help you lose weight more quickly. Why? Because the more active you are, the more calories you will burn.

4 The long and the short

If you are pushed for time, take a shorter walk instead. Researchers at Loughborough University found that women walking for 30 minutes five days a week had almost identical fitness to those who split it into three longer stints.

5 Keep an exercise diary

Add exercise notes to your daily food diary to help keep you motivated to walk or work out every day.

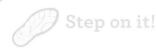

Step on it!

Get fresh air
People who walked, hiked or biked on trails at least once a week were twice as likely to get 30 minutes of exercise almost every day as those who didn't head outdoors, researchers at the University of Utah found.

Fact or fiction?

✘ FICTION: You can spot-reduce to lose weight.

✔ FACT: Working all the muscles gets results.

The way to achieve sleeker legs or a flatter stomach, if that's where you're carrying your body fat, is to increase your lean muscle tissue throughout your body. By working all your muscles, you increase your metabolism. Increase your metabolism and watch your eating, then you'll start looking the way you want to.

TONE UP AT HOME

You don't have to go to a gym to get fit. Combine these four exercises to create a mini exercise circuit. Do each exercise for 40 seconds with a 20-second break in between, and repeat each exercise three to four times. Do the circuit three times a week and you'll soon see the difference.

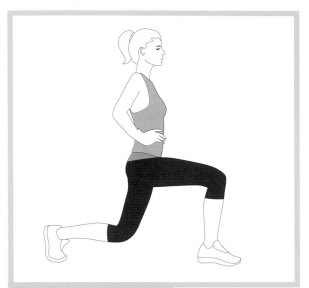

Lunges to tone your legs and bottom

Stand with your feet shoulder-width apart. Take a large step backwards with your right leg as you bend your left leg and lower your hips. Lower yourself into a one-legged squat position on your left leg, until your left thigh is parallel to the floor. Hold for a second, then push hard through your left leg to return to the starting position. Keep your body erect throughout the movement – do not lean forwards. Alternate with the left leg leading.

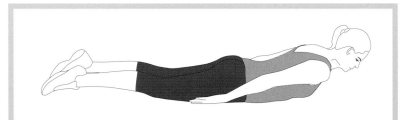

Back extension

Lie face down with your arms behind your back. Slowly raise your head, shoulders and upper chest from the floor. This will be just a short distance. Pause for a count of two, then lower slowly to the floor. Keep your head facing downwards in line with your spine. This will strengthen your back and improve your posture.

Half press-ups for shaping the chest and arms

Lie on the floor, face down, resting your weight on your knees. Place your hands slightly wider than shoulder-width apart under your shoulders, fingers pointing forwards. Keeping a straight line through your torso, bend your arms until your nose almost touches the floor. Aim your chest between your hands. Straighten your arms back to the start position.

 Step on it!

Working all the muscles gets results
The way to achieve sleeker legs or a flatter stomach, if that's where you're carrying your fat, lean muscle tissue throughout your body. By working all your muscles, you increase your metabolism. Increase your metabolism and watch your eating, then you'll start looking the way you want to.

Plank for a flat tummy

Lie face down with your hands either side of your head and your elbows on the ground. Push yourself up, keeping your weight on your forearms and toes. Your elbows should be bent at 90°. Keep your back straight – your head, back, hips and ankles should be in a straight line. Hold and then slowly lower yourself back to the start position.

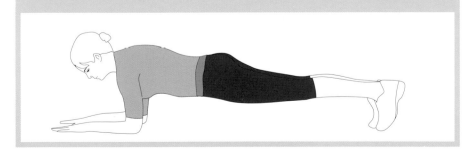

FAT-BUSTING WEEKDAY MEAL PLANNER

	MONDAY	TUESDAY	WEDNESDAY	THURSDAY	FRIDAY
BREAKFAST (about 350 calories)	1 x 125g pot low-fat yogurt with 3 tbsp granola and 1 grated apple	2 Oatibix with 250ml (9fl oz) skimmed milk and 1 tbsp chopped nuts or seeds; 1 orange	Berry smoothie (whizz handful of berries with 1 x 125ml pot low-fat yogurt and 275ml skimmed milk); 20g (¾oz) nuts	2 slices of wholemeal toast with 2 tsp butter and 1 boiled egg	Porridge made with 40g (1½oz) oats, 250ml (9fl oz) skimmed milk; 1 banana
LUNCH (about 500 calories)	Mozzarella, avocado and tomato salad (50g /2oz mozzarella with ½ sliced avocado, 1 sliced tomato and 1 tbsp oil/ balsamic dressing) with 1 slice wholemeal bread	Carrot and Sweet Potato Soup (p. 137) with 1 wholemeal roll, 2 tsp butter and 2 tbsp grated cheese	Orange and Chicken Salad (p. 138) with 1 slice wholemeal bread and 2 tsp butter	200g (7oz) baked beans with 1 medium baked potato; 1 x 125g (4oz) low-fat yogurt and 1 pear	50g (2oz) goat's cheese with leafy salad and 1 tbsp oil/ vinegar dressing; 1 x 175g pot fat-free Greek yogurt with honey
DINNER (about 500 calories)	Pappardelle with Spinach (p. 133); 150g (5oz) strawberries	125g (4oz) cubed lean lamb fillet kebabs served with 50g (2oz) flatbread and a tomato/ cucumber/olive salad	Butternut Squash and Spinach Lasagne (p. 133) and a mixed salad with 1 tbsp oil/vinegar dressing; 125g (4oz) fruit salad	Stir-fried veg (broccoli, mushrooms, pepper, courgettes) with 125g (4oz) prawns and 3 tbsp rice; ¼ cantaloupe melon	Sardines with Mediterranean Vegetables (p. 131) plus 100g (3½oz) new potatoes
SNACK (about 100 calories)	½ mango and 100g (3½oz) grapes	1 Müller Light yogurt (any flavour)	1 rice cake with 1 tsp peanut butter	200g (7oz) fresh pineapple and melon	20g (¾oz) almonds or cashew nuts

Before you eat that biscuit, chocolate bar or bag of crisps, consider how long you'll have to exercise to work it off!

FOOD OR DRINK	TIME TO BURN IT OFF WALKING AT A MODERATE SPEED*
Cadbury's Dairy Milk chocolate 49g bar, 260 calories	76 minutes
Häagen-Dazs vanilla ice cream 100ml tub, 225 calories	70 minutes
Cola 330ml can, 135 calories	41 minutes
Apple juice 200ml (7fl oz) glass, 76 calories	23 minutes
Krispy Kreme glazed raspberry doughnut 86g (3¼oz) doughnut, 307 calories	92 minutes
Kettle chips 40g bag, 192 calories	58 minutes
Chocolate Hobnobs 2 biscuits, 184 calories	56 minutes
Starbucks coffee frappuccino grande, semi-skimmed, 232 calories	70 minutes
Starbucks classic blueberry muffin 1 muffin, 481 calories	144 minutes
Kit Kat 4 fingers, 233 calories	70 minutes
*Calculations based on a 63kg (10 stone) woman.	

Party time

You can celebrate good times without derailing your diet. Here's how to eat, drink, and enjoy a slice of cake – without piling on the pounds.

Party time often translates into eating time. In fact, celebrations are usually coupled with special foods – mince pies at Christmas, canapés and champagne at New Year – not to mention celebration cakes on birthdays, weddings and christenings! Merrymaking usually means rich foods – and reasons to share and indulge in them. Yet it's hard to munch on carrots when everyone else is enjoying canapés or cake. In order to enjoy celebrations and fit into that party dress for the next big event, you need to have a plan.

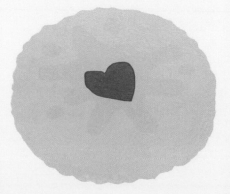

1 Get prepared

Before that birthday picnic, Christmas dinner or family get-together, recognize the situations that cause you to overindulge, then strategize. Mental rehearsal can help you to anticipate eating cues and how to respond to them. Spend a minute or two rehearsing your performance, preferably just before you enter the party. Then you'll know your line of attack (have just a small piece of cake and only one cocktail, for example) when you enter the dieting danger zone.

2 Be a picky eater

Think of the calories you'll eat as money in the bank: make wise investments with your calories, selecting the best of the offerings and passing up foods that are available anytime. (Auntie Mary's world-famous lemon meringue pie is worth every calorie; a bowl of crisps is not.) Select your favourite special foods to splurge on and eat one or two, not the entire tray.

3 Keep moving

Exercise burns calories and helps you control your weight – but only if you work out on a regular basis. During the festive season and while on holiday, it's tempting to abandon your exercise routine, but in truth, this is the worst time to skimp. Every week, try to have as many 'normal' days – when you eat healthy foods and exercise – as possible.

If it's just impossible to take an exercise break, think of other ways you can be active. Even if you're not challenging your body with your usual workout, there are other ways to burn a few extra calories. If you're at a party, volunteer to clear the tables or fetch items from the kitchen; if you're at a family gathering, take 20 minutes to play chase with your nieces and nephews. When you're on holiday, go for walks.

4 Make peace with your cravings

A Drexel University study found that people who had been taught to use techniques similar to mindfulness meditation (accepting that thoughts are just thoughts and don't require a rush to judgement or action) were better able to resist a treat – in this case, a packet of biscuits – than those who didn't have the training. 'If you try to make your cravings go away, all your focus is on the food', says researcher Evan Forman. 'But if you just exist with the thought, it loses its power.' One way to make that easier is to take a moment to think about what you want out of life, which feeding your craving might deny you. To be fit enough to play with your kids? Slim enough to wear a slinky red dress to your New Year's Eve party? 'Identifying what's ultimately important to you will allow that goal – rather than a food craving – to direct your behaviour', says Forman.

5 Drop the all-or-nothing attitude

'I blew it at lunch, so I might as well pig out at dinner.' All right, you had a celebratory lunch with a few friends, or perhaps you drank three jumbo-sized cocktails at a party or ordered an appetizer and shared a dessert on a special evening out. All told, you've taken in an extra 500–600 calories for the day. If you then take a no-holds-barred approach to your next meal, you risk turning that 500–600-calorie infraction into a 1,500–1,600-calorie debacle. Don't beat yourself up. If you do overindulge, acknowledge that you feel bad about it, but use that energy to redouble your efforts – shift your mindset from 'I am a failure' to 'I'm back on track!'

Whether it's a birthday bash, a family gathering or an office get-together, here's how to enjoy the party while keeping your weight-loss goal in mind.

1 Don't arrive ravenous
Before leaving home, eat a little protein-packed snack such as yogurt, cottage cheese, a few nuts, turkey or chicken. This way, you'll have more resistance when you face tempting calorific fare.

2 Portion control
You can eat what you love, just not a lot of it. You'll feel more satisfied indulging in a small portion of lasagne, say, than eating just vegetables (see also page 56).

3 Pick your pleasures
Choose the three to five dishes that are the most appealing. Fill your plate with

Diet trap
MISBEHAVING AT THE BUFFET
In a study by Cornell University's Food and Brand lab, 22 trained spectators watched 213 diners at 11 all-you-can eat Chinese food buffets in several cities. Patrons who were overweight or obese were more likely than normal-weight patrons to:
• Serve themselves immediately (rather than scan buffet options).
• Choose a large plate.
• Sit facing the buffet.
• Sit without a napkin on their laps.
If you're dining at an all-you-can eat buffet and watching your weight, face away from the buffet, use a small plate and browse choices before you load your plate. The napkin is up to you!

Swap this:
338 calories for 100g (3½oz) strawberry cheesecake
For this:
183 calories for 125g (4oz) (about 10) strawberries with 2 tbsp double cream

small tastes of these, skip the other buffet items (or fill the rest of your plate with vegetables or leafy salad), and don't go back for more.

4 Check your hunger
Often, the desire to eat is not about hunger but rather about how delicious the food tastes. If you're satisfied, don't automatically reach for a second sausage roll or another slice of cake.

5 Take a seat
When you're standing and chatting while eating, it's difficult to keep tabs on how much you're consuming. If possible, sit down at a table and be mindful of what you are eating.

A traditional Christmas lunch with all the trimmings can pack a hefty 1,000 calories. Use the tactics below for your favourite Christmas dishes and you can save loads of calories.

DIET MADNESS	DIET MAKEOVER	YOU SAVE
Brandy butter, 1 tbsp *225 calories*	Brandy custard, 2 tbsp *109 calories*	*116 calories*
Bread sauce, 2 tbsp *100 calories*	Cranberry sauce, 1 heaped tbsp *45 calories*	*55 calories*
2 bacon-wrapped sausages *240 calories*	½ rasher of bacon around a mini reduced-fat sausage *40 calories*	*200 calories*
Roast turkey leg meat with skin, 150g (5oz) *266 calories*	Turkey breast meat without skin, 150g (5oz) *140 calories*	*126 calories*
Buttered carrots and Brussels sprouts, 150g (5oz) *157 calories*	Boiled carrots and Brussels sprouts, 150g (5oz) *45 calories*	*112 calories*
Mince pie with 1 tbsp brandy butter *464 calories*	Mince pie with 1 tbsp single cream *268 calories*	*196 calories*
3 roast potatoes *381 calories*	150g (5oz) swede, carrots and parsnips roasted with 1 tsp oil *177 calories*	*204 calories*

Although Christmas is notoriously dangerous for diets, summer celebrations and barbecues can also be calorie minefields. Barbecues don't have to spell trouble for your waistline. These tips can help you eat healthily but still savour the flavours.

1 Go skin-free and low-fat

Grill skinless chicken, seafood and lean cuts of beef, pork or lamb, not high-fat hot dogs, hamburgers and sausages.

2 Add calorie-free flavour

Use flavoured wood chips (like mesquite or apple wood) with coals to give food a nice smoky accent.

3 Pre-treat the meat

For tender, delicious chicken, marinate it in plain low-fat yogurt and mint; soak steak in soy sauce with fresh garlic. Try a 'dry rub': mix spices and herbs and rub them on meat, poultry or fish before grilling. Or brush on low-fat salad dressing during grilling to keep fish and fresh vegetables moist.

4 Eat your vegetables

Load up on grilled corn on the cob, aubergine, courgettes, mushrooms, peppers and other fresh vegetables.

5 Don't forget dessert

Grill cinnamon-dusted peach halves or pineapple wedges sprinkled with powdered ginger.

Swap this
337 calories for a 125g (4oz) barbecued spare rib
For this
123 calories for a 125g (4oz) barbecued lean pork kebab

Swap this
289 calories for 125g (4oz) potato salad
For this
187 calories for a 150g (5oz) baked potato with 10g (¼oz) butter

Swap this
214 calories for 1 handful, 35g (1¼oz), tortilla chips with 20g (¾oz) (about 1 tbsp) soured cream and chive dip
For this
105 calories for 10 mini breadsticks with 50g (2oz) (about 1 tbsp) tomato salsa

Birthdays, weddings, christenings and lots of other celebratory occasions go hand-in-hand with calorie-rich cake. But no food is so high in fat or sugar that eating it occasionally is going to ruin your Drop a Dress Size efforts.

Cake, just like doughnuts, pastries, chocolate and other weight-loss saboteurs, can be part of your diet as long as you can make it fit within your daily calorie budget. This means eating less before or after consuming the cake, having just a small slice or a few bites, or upping your activity to burn off the extra calories. If it's your celebration, try serving small cupcakes instead of a traditional cake.

Nibble on this

Need some motivation to stop at just one or two canapés? Take a look at how easily a few bites can add up:

- 2 handfuls of tortilla chips = 130 calories
- 1 mini sausage roll = 200 calories
- 2 slices of garlic bread = 200 calories
- 1 mini samosa = 150 calories
- 1 smoked salmon blini = 120 calories

Simple
swaps

Swap this
356 calories for a
125g (4oz) serving of
tiramisu
For this
231 calories
125g (4oz) serving of
raspberry mousse

It's not just about the food

Here are some more strategies for how to avoid the temptations of high-calorie fare:

- Wear a figure-hugging outfit, with a belt if possible. The snug fit will remind you not to stuff yourself to discomfort.
- Make socializing, rather than food, the focus of the event. Decide ahead of time that you will learn something new about someone you don't know well at the party.
- Put a special piece of jewellery on your hand or arm – a sparkly bangle or a big ring, for example – as a visible reminder to eat in moderation.
- Practise saying 'No, thank you', or stall with 'Not just yet'. It's OK to turn down a rich dessert or tell an eager host that you don't want seconds.

Pie

If you're craving apple pie (at 411 calories per 150g slice), try this simple recipe for cinnamon apple instead (a mere 115 calories per portion):

Core a cooking apple and peel one-third of the way down. Sprinkle the top with cinnamon, grated nutmeg and 1 tsp brown sugar. Cook in the microwave, covered, on medium power for 2–3 minutes, or until tender. You'll save 295 calories.

- Removing the icing and marzipan from a slice of Christmas cake will save about 150 calories.
- Two chocolate Brazil nuts = five After Eight mints = 200 calories

It pays to be prepared for festivities to avoid the disappointment of putting on extra weight. According to a study from the National Institutes of Health, the fabled festive season weight gain (from Christmas to New Year) is no myth. While the pounds added were modest (about one each year), that weight tends to stay on and accumulate over time. Here's how to prevent that happening.

Crunch time

Christmas shopping may trim your wallet, but it could also flatten your belly. As you search store shelves, stand tall and squeeze your stomach muscles for five seconds (pretend you're bracing yourself to lift a heavy box). Ta-da! You've done the equivalent of one sit-up.

Deal with seasonal stress

It's easy to underestimate the toll Christmas takes – physically, psychologically and emotionally. You may be feeling financially pinched or extra tired from lack of sleep, and extended visits with your family are not always tension-free. To avoid using eating as an emotional crutch, try these strategies for basic self-preservation.

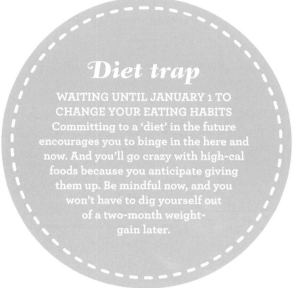

Diet trap

WAITING UNTIL JANUARY 1 TO CHANGE YOUR EATING HABITS Committing to a 'diet' in the future encourages you to binge in the here and now. And you'll go crazy with high-cal foods because you anticipate giving them up. Be mindful now, and you won't have to dig yourself out of a two-month weight-gain later.

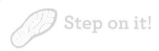

Step on it!

Chew gum while you tidy the kitchen
During the post-party kitchen clean-up, chew a piece of sugar-free gum to stop yourself snacking on leftovers. You can add a few hundred calories just by grazing on those last few bites.

Take a quick walk A California State University study that tracked frequent emotional snackers found that those who went for a brisk five-minute walk when they felt frazzled were much less likely to eat than those who just sat still.

Don't get caught up in the festive frenzy If there are too many parties, decline a few. If all the shopping stress is causing you to overeat, talk to your family about ways to make this year less chaotic. The more open and honest you are with yourself and with family and friends, the less likely it is that you'll turn to food to soothe yourself during the season.

Buddy-up to manage stress To avoid gaining weight now, you need commitment and awareness. It's best to work on both with a group of people – or even one or two close friends – whom you can call when an emotionally triggered eating craving strikes. So instead of polishing off a carton of ice cream after a stressful family dinner, phone a friend to share how you feel and then deal with the emotions.

Write it down

You've already learned, in Eating In (pages 14–35), about the importance of keeping a food diary. This is even more crucial during the festive period, when you'll be tempted with foods you might not normally eat (baking a dozen mince pies on a random Sunday would be crazy, but at Christmastime, it's practically required). Research has shown that writing everything down helps successful dieters lose weight and keep it off – more than anything else. It's the willingness to pay attention to what you're eating that's critical.

Swap this
270 calories for 5 mini Scotch eggs

For this
156 calories for 125g (4oz) mixed antipasti (mixed veg in olive oil)

Keep tabs on alcoholic drinks: they're often loaded with calories – especially the fancy concoctions. Even worse, alcohol lowers your inhibitions, making it more likely you'll go back for seconds (or thirds). That's why we suggest a 150-calorie cut-off. To see how quickly the calories from alcohol add up, consult the chart.

DRINK	CALORIES
Alcohol-free wine, per 175ml (6fl oz) glass	35
Bacardi Breezer, per 275ml (9½fl oz) glass	196
Bailey's, per 50ml (2fl oz) glass	160
Beer, per 300ml (½ pint) glass	96
Brandy, per single, 25ml (1fl oz) glass	56
Buck's fizz, per 175 ml (6fl oz) glass	105
Champagne, per 175ml (6fl oz) glass	133
Cider, dry, per 300ml (½ pint) glass	108
Drambuie, per single, 25ml (1fl oz) glass	79
Gin and tonic, per 250ml can	180
Guinness, per 300ml (½ pint) glass	90
Lager, per 300ml (½ pint) glass	87
Martini and lemonade, per 200ml (7fl oz) glass	91
Mulled wine, per 200ml (7fl oz) glass	210
Pimm's and lemonade, per 250ml can	161

Note: calorie counts may vary slightly depending on proportions of ingredients used.

DRINK	CALORIES
Piña colada, per 200ml (7fl oz) glass	185
Port, per 50ml (2fl oz) glass	78
Red wine, per 175ml (6fl oz) glass	119
Rosé wine, per 175ml (6fl oz) glass	124
Sangria, per 200ml (7fl oz) glass	200
Sherry, dry, per 50ml (2fl oz) glass	58
Sparkling wine, per 175ml (6fl oz) glass	130
Tequila, per 37.5ml (1.3fl oz) shot	99
Vodka and Coke, per 250ml (9fl oz) glass	132
Vodka and Diet Coke, per 250ml (9fl oz) glass	50
Vodka and slimline tonic, per 250ml (9fl oz) glass	50
White wine (dry), per 175ml (6fl oz) glass	115
White wine, medium, per 175ml (6fl oz) glass	130
White wine, sweet, per 175ml (6fl oz) glass	165

Note: calorie counts may vary slightly depending on proportions of ingredients used.

This flat-tummy plan will help you get into shape for the party season. Follow this series of exercises to get a slimmer waist and improve your posture.

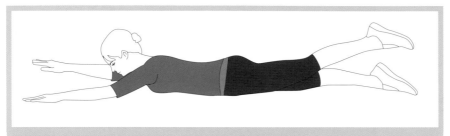

Superman

Lie on your front with your arms stretched in front of you. Lift your right arm and your left leg off the floor, keeping your head on the floor. Hold this position for a second. Lower slowly and repeat with the left arm and right leg. Repeat 10 times, alternating between left and right.

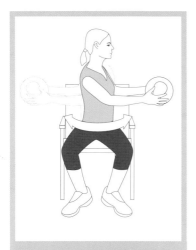

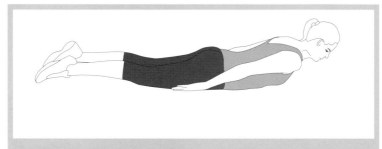

Back extensions

Lie face down on the floor with your arms by your sides. Raise your head, shoulders and upper chest from the floor. Hold for a second and squeeze the shoulder blades together, then lower slowly to the floor. Repeat 12–15 times.

Seated twist

Sit on a stability/Swiss ball or chair and hold a medicine ball (or medium-sized ball) close to your chest. Rotate your body to the right and then to the left. Perform in a smooth, continuous motion. Repeat 10–12 times.

Crunches

Lie on your back with your hands by your ears. Bend your legs and keep your feet flat on the floor. Raise your shoulders about 5cm (2in) off the ground. Hold for a second, then lower them back to the starting position. Keep your lower back on the floor throughout the move. Repeat 12–15 times.

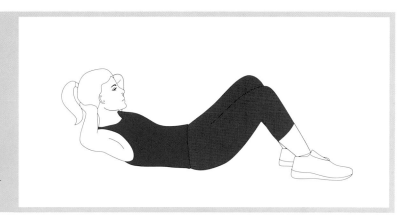

Toe taps

Lie back and support your upper body on your elbows and forearms. Keep your knees bent and lift your feet off the floor so that your lower legs are parallel to the floor. This is the starting position. Lower your feet to the floor until your toes touch, then return to the starting position. Repeat 12–15 times.

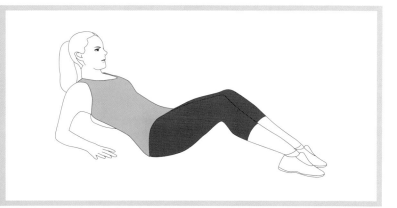

Cycling

Lie on your back with your hands by your ears and your legs raised, knees bent at a 90° angle. Raise your head and shoulders. Bring your left elbow towards your right knee while extending your left leg. Repeat on the other side. Repeat 12–15 times, alternating between left and right.

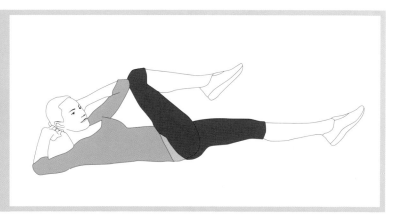

FAT-BUSTING WEEKDAY MEAL PLANNER

	MONDAY	TUESDAY	WEDNESDAY	THURSDAY	FRIDAY
BREAKFAST (about 350 calories)	2 Weetabix with 250ml (9fl oz) skimmed milk; 1 x 125g pot Activia yogurt	Porridge made with 40g (1½oz) oats, 250ml (9fl oz) skimmed milk and a little cinnamon; 25g (1oz) sultanas	1 Innocent mango and passionfruit smoothie; 20g (¾oz) nuts	40g (1½oz) Oats 'N' More, with 1 banana, 1 tbsp seeds and 125ml (4fl oz) skimmed milk	1 slice of wholemeal toast with 1 tsp butter and 1 poached egg; 3 tbsp baked beans
LUNCH (about 500 calories)	½ carton, 300ml (½ pint), New Covent Garden spicy butternut squash and sweet potato soup; 1 wholemeal roll with 1 tsp butter; 1 orange	Smoked Mackerel Citrus Salad (p. 138); 1 slice of wholemeal bread with 1 tsp butter; 2 plums	Turkey and salad wholemeal sandwich; 150g (5oz) fruit salad	Tuna salad (p. 137) with 1 wholemeal roll and 2 tsp butter; 1 x 125ml pot low-fat yogurt	2-egg omelette with tomatoes and 1 tbsp cheese; leafy salad with 1 tbsp oil and vinegar dressing; 1 nectarine
DINNER (about 500 calories)	One-pan Chicken with Tomatoes (p. 139), 200g (7oz) jacket potato with 2 tsp butter; leafy salad	Roasted Stuffed Peppers (p. 135); 3 tbsp wholegrain rice with broccoli; 150g (5oz) fruit salad	Pumpkin with Chickpeas (p. 135); 200g (7oz) new potatoes; cabbage	1 grilled skinless chicken breast; 200g (7oz) jacket potato with 2 tsp butter; carrots and green beans; 150g (5oz) fruit salad	Pork and Noodle Stir-fry (p. 140)
SNACK (about 100 calories)	1 pear and 100g (3½oz) grapes	1 wholegrain crispbread with 15g (½oz) Cheddar cheese	20g (¾oz) mixed seeds	Danone Shape Delights fat-free yogurt	20g (¾oz) nuts

BE A LONG-TERM LOSER

Build these simple habits into your life to keep your weight steady for a lifetime:

• Remember why you wanted to lose weight. Go back to your list (see page 000).
• Celebrate success. Small changes can make a big impact, so reward yourself with a manicure or a trip to the theatre or a show!
• Change the way you think about food. Instead of 'That chocolate bar looks good', think 'If I don't eat that, I'll feel better about myself.'
• Get professional support. See your GP and ask to be referred to a dietician. Or visit www.dietitiansunlimited.co.uk.
• Find an online weight-loss buddy. A study found an online buddy help you to keep weight off better than a face-to-face buddy. See www.weightlossresources.co.uk/weight_loss/weight-loss-buddy.htm
• Use your social network! Telling others about your goal really does help.
• Spring-clean your wardrobe. Be ruthless and get rid of 'fat' clothes.

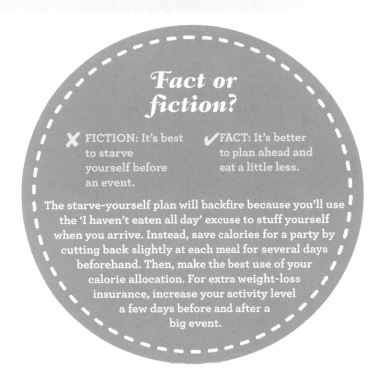

Fact or fiction?

✗ FICTION: It's best to starve yourself before an event.

✓ FACT: It's better to plan ahead and eat a little less.

The starve-yourself plan will backfire because you'll use the 'I haven't eaten all day' excuse to stuff yourself when you arrive. Instead, save calories for a party by cutting back slightly at each meal for several days beforehand. Then, make the best use of your calorie allocation. For extra weight-loss insurance, increase your activity level a few days before and after a big event.

The recipes

Here you'll find all the healthy recipes featured in the Weekday Meal Planners at the end of each chapter. These delicious and easy-to-prepare recipes will help you keep within your Drop A Dress Size daily targets. They are low in calories, saturated fat and crammed with vitamins and minerals.

All have been triple-tested in the Good Housekeeping dedicated kitchens so they are guaranteed to succeed. They emphasise everyday, healthy ingredients such fresh veggies, lean meat, poultry, oily fish, beans and herbs, all of which are widely available in supermarkets. Healthy cooking need not be time-consuming – most of the recipes in this section take less than 20 minutes to prepare. They make enough for at least 4 servings so you can add them to your repertoire of family meals.

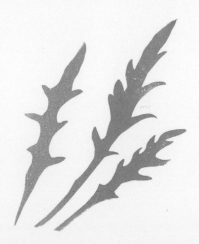

Chicken Stir-fry with Noodles

SERVES 4

250g pack thick egg noodles
2 tbsp vegetable oil
2 garlic cloves, crushed
4 boneless, skinless chicken breasts, each sliced into 10 pieces
3 medium carrots, about 450g (1lb), cut into thin strips about 5cm (2in) long
1 bunch of spring onions, sliced
200g (7oz) mangetouts
155g jar sweet chilli and lemongrass sauce

1 Cook the noodles in boiling water according to the pack instructions.
2 Meanwhile, heat the oil in a wok or frying pan. Add the garlic and stir-fry for 1–2 minutes. Add the chicken pieces and stir-fry for 5 minutes, then add the carrot strips and stir-fry for a further 5 minutes.
3 Add the spring onions, mangetouts and sauce to the wok and stir-fry for 5 minutes.
4 Drain the cooked noodles well and add to the wok. Toss everything together and serve.

Preparation Time: 20 minutes
Cooking Time: 20 minutes
Per Serving: 355 calories, 10g fat (of which 2g saturates), 29g carbohydrate, 0.5g salt

Dairy free

Grilled Spicy Chicken

SERVES 4

4 boneless, skinless chicken breasts
1 tbsp coriander seeds, crushed
1 tsp ground cumin
2 tsp mild curry paste
1 garlic clove, crushed
450g (1lb) natural yogurt
3 tbsp freshly chopped coriander
salt and ground black pepper
fresh coriander sprigs to garnish
mixed salad and rice to serve

1 Prick the chicken breasts all over with a fork, cover with clingfilm and beat lightly with a rolling pin to flatten them slightly.
2 Mix the coriander seeds with the cumin, curry paste, garlic and yogurt in a large shallow dish. Season with salt and pepper, and stir in the chopped coriander.
3 Add the chicken and turn to coat with the spiced yogurt. Cover and leave to marinate in the fridge for at least 30 minutes or overnight.
4 Preheat the barbecue or griddle. Lift the chicken out of the marinade and cook over a medium-high heat, turning occasionally, for about 20 minutes or until cooked through. Serve immediately, with rice and a mixed salad, garnished with coriander sprigs.

Preparation Time: 10 minutes, plus marinating
Cooking Time: About 20 minutes
Per Serving: 157 calories, 2g fat (of which 1g saturates), 3g carbohydrate, 0.2g salt

Gluten free

Sardines with Mediterranean Vegetables

SERVES 4

3 tbsp olive oil
2 red onions, about 300g (11oz), halved and cut into petals
2 garlic cloves, crushed
2 red peppers, about 375g (12oz), seeded and cut into chunks
225g (8oz) courgettes, cut into small chunks
900g (2lb) sardines (about 16), cleaned
olive oil and lemon juice to drizzle
salt and ground black pepper
small fresh basil sprigs to garnish

1 Heat the oil in a large griddle, or preheat the grill. Add the onions and fry for 2–3 minutes until almost soft. Add the garlic and peppers and stir-fry for 5 minutes, then add the courgettes and stir-fry for 4–5 minutes until almost soft. Remove from the griddle and keep warm.
2 Season the sardines and cook on the griddle or under the hot grill for 3–4 minutes on each side, until cooked in the centre.
3 Drizzle the sardines with a little olive oil and lemon juice. Garnish with basil sprigs and serve with the vegetables.

Preparation Time: **15 minutes**
Cooking Time: **20 minutes**
Per Serving: **409 calories, 23g fat (of which 5g saturates), 13g carbohydrate, 0.5g salt**

Gluten free
Dairy free

Cod with Cherry Tomatoes

SERVES 4

4 × 100g (3½oz) cod steaks
1 tbsp plain flour
2 tbsp olive oil
1 small onion, sliced
1 large red chilli, seeded and chopped
1 garlic clove, crushed
250g (9oz) cherry tomatoes, halved
4 spring onions, chopped
2 tbsp freshly chopped coriander
salt and ground black pepper

1 Season the cod with salt and pepper, then dust lightly with the flour. Heat 1 tbsp oil in a large frying pan. Add the onion and fry for 5–10 minutes until golden.
2 Pour the remaining oil into the pan. Add the cod and fry for 3 minutes on each side. Add the chilli, garlic, cherry tomatoes, spring onions and coriander, and season with salt and pepper. Cover and continue to cook for 5–10 minutes until everything is heated through. Serve immediately.

Preparation Time: **15 minutes**
Cooking Time: **20–25 minutes**
Per Serving: **168 calories, 7g fat (of which 1g saturates), 8g carbohydrate, 0.2g salt**

Dairy free

Classic Lasagne

SERVES
6

butter to grease
350g (12oz) fresh lasagne, or 225g (8oz) 'no need to pre-cook' lasagne (12–15 sheets)
3 tbsp freshly grated Parmesan
mixed salad leaves to serve

For the bolognese sauce
2 tbsp olive oil
1 onion, finely chopped
2 garlic cloves, crushed
450g (1lb) extra-lean minced beef
2 tbsp sun-dried tomato paste
300ml (½ pint) red wine
400g can chopped tomatoes
125g (4oz) chestnut mushrooms, sliced
2 tbsp Worcestershire sauce
salt and ground black pepper
mixed salad leaves to serve

For the béchamel sauce
300ml (½ pint) semi-skimmed milk
1 onion slice
6 peppercorns
1 mace blade
1 bay leaf
15g (½oz) butter
15g (½oz) plain flour
freshly grated nutmeg
salt and ground black pepper

1 To make the bolognese sauce, heat the oil in a large pan, add the onion and fry over a medium heat for 10 minutes or until softened and golden. Add the garlic and cook for 1 minute. Add the beef and brown evenly, using a wooden spoon to break up the pieces. Stir in the tomato paste and wine, cover and bring to the boil. Add the tomatoes, mushrooms and Worcestershire sauce, and season well with salt and pepper. Bring back to the boil, reduce the heat and simmer for 20 minutes. (If using 'no need to pre-cook' lasagne, add a little extra stock or water to the sauce.)

2 To make the béchamel sauce, pour the milk into a pan and add the onion, peppercorns, mace and bay leaf. Bring almost to the boil, then remove from the heat, cover and leave to infuse for about 20 minutes. Strain. Melt the butter in a pan, stir in the flour and cook, stirring, for 1 minute or until cooked but not coloured. Remove from the heat and gradually pour in the milk, whisking constantly. Season lightly with nutmeg, salt and pepper. Put back on the heat and cook, stirring constantly, until the sauce is thickened and smooth. Simmer gently for 2 minutes.

3 Preheat the oven to 180°C (160°C fan oven) mark 4. Spoon one-third of the bolognese sauce over the base of a greased 2.3 litre (4 pint) ovenproof dish. Cover with a layer of lasagne sheets, then a layer of béchamel sauce. Repeat these layers twice more, finishing with a layer of béchamel sauce to cover the lasagne.

4 Sprinkle the Parmesan over the top and stand the dish on a baking sheet. Cook in the oven for 45 minutes, or until well browned and bubbling. Serve with mixed salad leaves.

Preparation Time: About 1 hour 20 minutes
Cooking Time: 45 minutes
Per Serving: 326 calories, 13g fat (of which 6g saturates), 37g carbohydrate, 0.5g salt

Pappardelle with Spinach

SERVES
4

350g (12oz) pappardelle
350g (12oz) baby leaf spinach, roughly chopped
2 tbsp olive oil
75g (3oz) ricotta cheese
freshly grated nutmeg
salt and ground black pepper

1 Cook the pappardelle in a large pan of boiling water, according to the pack instructions, until al dente.
2 Drain the pasta well, put back in the pan and add the spinach, oil and ricotta, tossing for 10–15 seconds until the spinach has wilted. Season with a little nutmeg, salt and pepper, and serve immediately.

Preparation Time: 5 minutes
Cooking Time: 12 minutes
Per Serving: 404 calories, 11g fat (of which 3g saturates), 67g carbohydrate, 0.3g salt

Vegetarian

Butternut Squash and Spinach Lasagne

SERVES
6

1 butternut squash, peeled, halved, seeded and cut into 3cm (1¼in) cubes
2 tbsp olive oil
1 onion, sliced
25g (1oz) butter
25g (1oz) plain flour
600ml (1 pint) milk
250g (9oz) ricotta cheese
1 tsp freshly grated nutmeg
225g bag baby leaf spinach
6 'no need to pre-cook' lasagne sheets
50g (2oz) pecorino cheese or Parmesan, freshly grated
salt and ground black pepper

1 Preheat the oven to 200°C (180°C fan oven) mark 6. Put the squash in a roasting tin with the oil, onion and 1 tbsp water. Mix; season. Roast for 25 minutes, tossing halfway through.
2 To make the sauce, melt the butter in a pan, stir in the flour and cook over a medium heat for 1–2 minutes. Gradually add the milk, stirring constantly. Reduce the heat and cook, stirring, for 5 minutes or until the sauce has thickened. Crumble in the ricotta; add the nutmeg. Mix together thoroughly and season.
3 Heat 1 tbsp water in a pan. Add the spinach, cover and cook until just wilted. Season well.
4 Spoon the squash mixture into a 1.7 litre (3 pint) ovenproof dish. Layer the spinach on top, then cover with one-third of the sauce, then the lasagne. Spoon the remaining sauce on top, season and sprinkle with the grated cheese. Cook for 30–35 minutes until the cheese topping is golden and the pasta cooked.

Preparation Time: 30 minutes
Cooking Time: About 1 hour
Per Serving: 273 calories, 17g fat (of which 7g saturates), 18g carbohydrate, 0.6g salt

Prawn and Vegetable Pilau

 SERVES 4

250g (9oz) long-grain rice
1 broccoli head, broken into florets
150g (5oz) baby sweetcorn, halved
200g (7oz) sugarsnap peas
1 red pepper, seeded and sliced into thin strips
400g (14oz) cooked and peeled king prawns

For the dressing
1 tbsp sesame oil
5cm (2in) piece fresh root ginger, peeled and grated
juice of 1 lime
1–2 tbsp light soy sauce

1 Put the rice into a large, wide pan – it needs to be really big, as you'll be cooking the rice and steaming the vegetables on top, then tossing it all together. Add 600ml (1 pint) boiling water. Cover and bring to the boil, then reduce the heat to low and cook the rice according to the pack instructions.
2 About 10 minutes before the end of the rice cooking time, add the broccoli, corn, sugarsnaps and red pepper. Stir well, then cover the pan and cook until the vegetables and rice are just tender.
3 Meanwhile, put the prawns into a bowl. Add the sesame oil, ginger, lime and soy sauce and stir well. Mix the prawns and dressing into the cooked vegetables and rice and toss well. Serve immediately.

Preparation Time: 10 minutes
Cooking Time: 15–20 minutes
Per Serving: 360 calories, 5g fat (of which 1g saturates), 61g carbohydrate, 1.8g salt

Dairy free

Tomato and Butter Bean Stew

 SERVES 6

2 tbsp olive oil
1 onion, finely sliced
2 garlic cloves, finely chopped
2 large leeks, trimmed and sliced
2 × 400g cans cherry tomatoes
2 × 400g cans butter beans with no added sugar or salt, drained and rinsed
150ml (¼ pint) hot vegetable stock
1–2 tbsp balsamic vinegar
salt and ground black pepper

1 Preheat the oven to 180°C (160°C fan oven) mark 4. Heat the oil in a flameproof casserole over a medium heat. Add the onion and garlic and cook for 10 minutes or until golden and soft. Add the leeks, cover and cook for 5 minutes.
2 Add the tomatoes, beans and hot stock, and season well with salt and pepper. Bring to the boil, then cover and cook in the oven for 35–40 minutes until the sauce has thickened. Remove from the oven, stir in the vinegar and spoon into warmed bowls.

Preparation Time: 10 minutes
Cooking Time: 50–55 minutes
Per Serving: 214 calories, 7g fat (of which 1g saturates), 29g carbohydrate, 0.2g salt

Vegetarian
Dairy free

Roasted Stuffed Peppers

SERVES 8

40g (1½oz) butter
4 Romano peppers, halved, with stalks on and seeded
3 tbsp olive oil
350g (12oz) chestnut mushrooms, roughly chopped
4 tbsp finely chopped fresh chives
100g (3½oz) vegetarian feta cheese
50g (2oz) fresh white breadcrumbs
25g (1oz) freshly grated Parmesan
salt and ground black pepper

1 Preheat the oven to 180°C (160°C fan oven) mark 4. Use a little of the butter to grease a shallow ovenproof dish and put the peppers in it side by side, ready to be filled.
2 Heat the remaining butter and 1 tbsp oil in a pan. Add the mushrooms and fry until they're golden and there's no excess liquid left in the pan. Stir in the chives, then spoon the mixture into the pepper halves.
3 Crumble the feta over the mushrooms. Mix the breadcrumbs and Parmesan in a bowl, then sprinkle over the peppers.
4 Season with salt and pepper, and drizzle with the remaining oil. Roast in the oven for 45 minutes or until golden and tender. Serve warm.

Preparation Time: 20 minutes
Cooking Time: 50 minutes
Per Serving: 189 calories, 14g fat (of which 6g saturates), 11g carbohydrate, 0.9g salt

Vegetarian

Pumpkin with Chickpeas

SERVES 6

900g (2lb) pumpkin or squash, such as butternut, Crown Prince or kabocha, peeled, seeded and chopped into roughly 2cm (¾in) cubes
1 garlic clove, crushed
2 tbsp olive oil
2 × 400g cans chickpeas, drained and rinsed
½ red onion, thinly sliced
1 large bunch of coriander, roughly chopped
salt and ground black pepper
steamed spinach to serve

For the tahini sauce
1 large garlic clove, crushed
3 tbsp tahini paste
juice of 1 lemon

1 Preheat the oven to 220°C (200°C fan oven) mark 7. Toss the squash or pumpkin in the garlic and oil, and season. Put in a roasting tin and roast for 25 minutes, or until soft.
2 Meanwhile, put the chickpeas into a pan with 150ml (¼ pint) water over a medium heat, to warm through.
3 To make the tahini sauce, put the garlic into a bowl, add a pinch of salt, then whisk in the tahini paste. Add the lemon juice and 4–5 tbsp cold water (consistency somewhere between single and double cream), then season to taste.
4 Put the chickpeas into a large bowl, then add the pumpkin, onion and coriander. Pour on the tahini sauce and toss carefully. Adjust the seasoning and serve while warm, with spinach.

Preparation Time: 15 minutes
Cooking Time: 25–30 minutes
Per Serving: 228 calories, 12g fat (of which 2g saturates), 22g carbohydrate, 0.6g salt

Vegetarian
Gluten free
Dairy free

Thai Vegetable Curry

SERVES 4

2–3 tbsp red Thai curry paste (suitable for vegetarians, if necessary)
2.5cm (1in) piece fresh root ginger, peeled and finely chopped
50g (2oz) cashew nuts
400ml can coconut milk
3 carrots, cut into thin batons
1 broccoli head, cut into florets
20g (¾oz) fresh coriander, roughly chopped
zest and juice of 1 lime
2 large handfuls of spinach leaves
basmati rice to serve

1 Put the curry paste into a large pan, add the ginger and cashew nuts and stir-fry over a medium heat for about 2–3 minutes.
2 Add the coconut milk, cover and bring to the boil. Stir the carrots into the pan, then reduce the heat and simmer for 5 minutes. Add the broccoli florets and simmer for a further 5 minutes until tender.
3 Stir the coriander and lime zest into the pan with the spinach. Squeeze the lime juice over the curry and serve with basmati rice.

Preparation Time: **10 minutes**
Cooking Time: **15 minutes**
Per Serving: **200 calories, 10g fat (of which 2g saturates), 19g carbohydrate, 0.7g salt**

Vegetarian
Gluten free
Dairy free

Summer Couscous

SERVES 4

175g (6oz) baby plum tomatoes, halved
2 small aubergines, thickly sliced
2 large yellow peppers, seeded and roughly chopped
2 red onions, cut into thin wedges
2 fat garlic cloves, crushed
5 tbsp olive oil
250g (9oz) couscous
400g can chopped tomatoes
2 tbsp harissa paste
25g (1oz) toasted pumpkin seeds (optional)
1 large bunch of coriander, roughly chopped
salt and ground black pepper

1 Preheat the oven to 230°C (210°C fan oven) mark 8. Put the vegetables and garlic into a large roasting tin, drizzle 3 tbsp oil over them and season with salt and pepper. Toss to coat. Roast for 20 minutes or until tender.
2 Meanwhile, put the couscous into a separate roasting tin and add 300ml (½ pint) cold water. Leave to soak for 5 minutes. Stir in the tomatoes and harissa and drizzle with the remaining oil. Put in the oven next to the vegetables for 4–5 minutes to warm through.
3 Stir the pumpkin seeds, if using, and the coriander into the couscous and season. Add the vegetables and stir.

Preparation Time: **10 minutes**
Cooking Time: **20 minutes**
Per Serving: **405 calories, 21g fat (of which 3g saturates), 49g carbohydrate, 0g salt**

Vegetarian
Dairy free

Tuna Salad

SERVES
4

2 × 400g cans mixed beans, drained and rinsed
250g (9oz) flaked tuna
1 cucumber, chopped
1 large red onion, finely sliced
4 ripe tomatoes, chopped
4 celery sticks, chopped
80g bag baby spinach leaves
2 tbsp olive oil
1 tsp red wine vinegar
salt and ground black pepper

1 Put the beans into a bowl and add the tuna,
cucumber, red onion, tomatoes, celery and
spinach.
2 Mix the oil and vinegar together, season with
salt and pepper, then toss the bean mix in the
dressing and serve immediately.

Preparation Time: **10 minutes**
Per Serving: **157 calories, 4g fat (of which trace
saturates), 9g carbohydrate, 0.5g salt**

Dairy free
Gluten free

Carrot and Sweet Potato Soup

SERVES
8

1 tbsp olive oil
1 large onion, chopped
1 tbsp coriander seeds
900g (2lb) carrots, roughly chopped
2 medium sweet potatoes, roughly chopped
2 litres (3½ pints) hot vegetable or chicken stock
2 tbsp white wine vinegar
2 tbsp freshly chopped coriander, plus extra
coriander leaves to garnish
4 tbsp half-fat crème fraîche
salt and ground black pepper

1 Heat the oil in a large pan. Add the onion and
coriander seeds and cook over a medium heat
for 5 minutes. Add the carrots and sweet
potatoes and cook for a further 5 minutes.
2 Add the hot stock and bring to the boil, then
reduce the heat and simmer for 25 minutes or
until the vegetables are tender.
3 Leave the soup to cool a little, then whizz in
batches in a blender or food processor until just
slightly chunky. Add the wine vinegar and
season with salt and pepper.
4 Pour the soup into a clean pan, stir in the
chopped coriander and reheat gently.
5 Drizzle the crème fraîche over it and sprinkle
with the coriander leaves. Serve in
warmed bowls.

Preparation Time: **15 minutes**
Cooking Time: **45 minutes**
Per Serving: **120 calories, 3g fat (of which 1g saturates),
22g carbohydrate, 0.7g salt**

Vegetarian
Gluten free

Orange and Chicken Salad

50g (2oz) cashew nuts
zest and juice of 2 oranges
2 tbsp marmalade
1 tbsp honey
1 tbsp oyster sauce
400g (14oz) roast chicken, shredded
a handful of chopped raw vegetables, such as
cucumber, carrot, red and yellow pepper and
Chinese leaves

1 Put the cashew nuts into a dry frying pan over
a medium-high heat and cook for 2–3 minutes,
tossing regularly, until golden brown. Tip into a
large serving bowl.
2 To make the dressing, put the orange zest
and juice into the frying pan with the
marmalade, honey and oyster sauce. Bring to
the boil, stirring, then simmer for about 2–3
minutes until slightly thickened.
3 Add the roast chicken to the serving bowl
with the chopped raw vegetables. Pour the
dressing over the salad, toss everything together
and serve immediately.

Preparation Time: **15 minutes**
Cooking Time: **10 minutes**
Per Serving: 252 calories, 8g fat (of which 2g saturates),
20g carbohydrate, 0.5g salt

Gluten free
Dairy free

Smoked Mackerel Citrus Salad

200g (7oz) green beans
200g (7oz) smoked mackerel fillets
125g (4oz) mixed watercress, spinach and rocket
4 spring onions, sliced
1 avocado, halved, stoned, peeled and sliced

For the dressing
1 tbsp olive oil
1 tbsp freshly chopped coriander
grated zest and juice of 1 orange

1 Preheat the grill. Blanch the green beans in
boiling water for 3 minutes until they are just
tender. Drain, rinse under cold running water,
drain well, then tip into a bowl.
2 Cook the mackerel under the hot grill for
2 minutes until warmed through. Flake into
bite-sized pieces, discard the skin and add the
fish to the bowl with the salad leaves, spring
onions and avocado.
3 Whisk all the dressing ingredients together in
a small bowl. Pour over the salad, toss well and
serve immediately.

Preparation Time: **10 minutes**
Cooking Time: **5 minutes**
Per Serving: 299 calories, 26g fat (of which 5g
saturates), 4g carbohydrate, 1g salt

Dairy free
Gluten free

Chickpea Curry

SERVES 6

2 tbsp vegetable oil
2 onions, finely sliced
2 garlic cloves, crushed
1 tbsp ground coriander
1 tsp mild chilli powder
1 tbsp black mustard seeds
2 tbsp tamarind paste
2 tbsp sun-dried tomato paste
750g (1lb 10oz) new potatoes, quartered
400g can chopped tomatoes
1 litre (1¾ pints) hot vegetable stock
250g (9oz) green beans, trimmed
2 × 400g cans chickpeas, drained and rinsed
2 tsp garam masala
salt and ground black pepper

1 Heat the oil in a pan and fry the onions for
10–15 minutes until golden. Add the garlic,
coriander, chilli, mustard seeds, tamarind paste
and sun-dried tomato paste. Cook for
1–2 minutes until the aroma from the spices
is released.
2 Add the potatoes and toss in the spices for
1–2 minutes. Add the tomatoes and hot stock;
season. Cover and bring to the boil. Simmer,
half-covered, for 20 minutes or until the
potatoes are just cooked.
3 Add the beans and chickpeas, and continue
to cook for 5 minutes or until the beans are
tender and the chickpeas are warmed through.
Stir in the garam masala and serve.

Preparation time 20 minutes
Cooking time 40–45 minutes
Per Serving: 291 calories, 8g fat (of which 1g
saturates), 46g carbohydrate, 1.3g salt

Vegetarian
Dairy free
Gluten free

One-pan Chicken with Tomatoes

SERVES 4

4 chicken thighs
1 red onion, sliced
400g can chopped tomatoes with herbs
400g can mixed beans
2 tsp balsamic vinegar
freshly chopped flat-leafed parsley to garnish

1 Heat a non-stick pan and fry the chicken
thighs, skin-side down, until golden. Turn over
and fry for 5 minutes.
2 Add the red onion and fry for 5 minutes. Add
the tomatoes, mixed beans and balsamic
vinegar. Cover and simmer for 10–12 minutes
until piping hot. Garnish with parsley and
serve immediately.

Preparation time 5 minutes
Cooking time 20–25 minutes
Per Serving: 238 calories, 4g fat (of which 1g saturates),
20g carbohydrate, 1g salt

Dairy free
Gluten free

Pork and Noodle Stir-fry

SERVES
4

1 tbsp sesame oil
5cm (2in) piece fresh root ginger, peeled and grated
2 tbsp soy sauce
1 tbsp fish sauce
½ red chilli, finely chopped
450g (1lb) stir-fry pork strips
2 red peppers, halved, seeded and roughly chopped
250g (9oz) baby sweetcorn, halved lengthways
200g (7oz) sugarsnap peas, halved
300g (11oz) bean sprouts
250g (9oz) rice noodles

1 Put the oil into a large bowl. Add the ginger, soy sauce, fish sauce, chilli and pork strips. Mix well and leave to marinate for 10 minutes.
2 Heat a large wok until hot. Lift the pork out of the marinade with a slotted spoon and add to the pan. Stir-fry over a high heat for 5 minutes. Add the red peppers, corn, sugarsnap peas, bean sprouts and remaining marinade, and stir-fry for a further 2–3 minutes until the pork is cooked.
3 Meanwhile, bring a large pan of water to the boil and cook the noodles according to the pack instructions.
4 Drain the noodles, tip into the wok and toss together, then serve immediately.

Preparation Time: **10 minutes, plus 10 minutes' marinating**
Cooking Time: **7–8 minutes**
Per Serving: **500 calories, 9g fat (of which 2g saturates), 67g carbohydrate, 3.4g salt**

Dairy free
Gluten free

Spiced Lamb with Lentils

SERVES
4

1 tbsp sunflower oil
8 lamb chops, trimmed of all fat
2 onions, finely sliced
1 tsp paprika
1 tsp ground cinnamon
400g can lentils, drained
400g can chickpeas, drained
300ml (½ pint) lamb or chicken stock
salt and ground black pepper
freshly chopped flat-leafed parsley to garnish

1 Preheat the oven to 180°C (160°C fan oven) mark 4. Heat the oil in a large, non-stick frying pan, add the chops and brown on both sides. Remove from the pan with a slotted spoon.
2 Add the onions, paprika and cinnamon. Fry for 2–3 minutes. Stir in the lentils and chickpeas. Season, then spoon into a shallow 2 litre (3½ pint) ovenproof dish.
3 Put the chops on top of the onion and lentil mixture and pour the stock over them.
4 Cover the dish tightly and cook in the oven for 1½ hours or until the chops are tender. Uncover and cook for 30 minutes or until lightly browned. Scatter over the parsley and serve hot.

Preparation Time: **10 minutes**
Cooking Time: **2 hours 10 minutes**
Per Serving: **315 calories, 12g fat (of which 2g saturates), 35g carbohydrate, 1g salt**

Dairy free
Gluten free

Turkey and Broccoli Stir-fry

SERVES 4

2 tbsp vegetable or sunflower oil
500g (1lb 2oz) turkey fillet, cut into strips
2 garlic cloves, crushed
2.5cm (1in) piece fresh root ginger, grated
1 broccoli head, chopped into florets
8 spring onions, finely chopped
125g (4oz) button mushrooms, halved
100g (3½oz) bean sprouts
3 tbsp oyster sauce
1 tbsp light soy sauce
125ml (4fl oz) hot chicken stock
juice of ½ lemon
egg noodles to serve

1 Heat 1 tbsp oil in a large, non-stick frying pan or wok, add the turkey strips and stir-fry for 4–5 minutes until golden and cooked through. Remove from the pan and set aside.
2 Heat the remaining oil in the same pan over a medium heat, add the garlic and ginger, and cook for 30 seconds, stirring all the time so that they don't burn. Add the broccoli, spring onions and mushrooms, turn up the heat and cook for 2–3 minutes until the vegetables start to brown but are still crisp.
3 Return the turkey to the pan and add the bean sprouts, sauces, hot stock and lemon juice. Cook for 1–2 minutes, tossing well to heat everything through, then serve with egg noodles.

Preparation Time: **15 minutes**
Cooking Time: **8–12 minutes**
Per Serving: **250 calories, 8g fat (of which 1g saturates), 7g carbohydrate, 1.2g salt**

Gluten free
Dairy free

Tomato, Pepper and Orange Soup

SERVES 4

3 rosemary sprigs
400g (14oz) jar roasted red peppers, drained
2 tsp golden caster sugar
1 litre (1¾ pints) tomato juice
4 very ripe plum tomatoes
300ml (½ pint) hot chicken stock
450ml (¾ pint) freshly squeezed orange juice
ground black pepper

1 Pull the leaves from the rosemary sprigs and discard the twiggy stalks. Put the leaves into a food processor or blender, add the peppers, sugar, half the tomato juice and the plum tomatoes and whizz together until just slightly chunky.
2 Sieve the mixture into a pan and stir in the stock, orange juice and the remaining tomato juice. Bring to the boil and simmer gently for about 10 minutes. Season with plenty of pepper to serve.

Preparation Time: **15 minutes**
Cooking Time: **12 minutes**
Per Serving: **136 calories, 1g fat (of which trace saturates), 30g carbohydrate, 1.8g salt**

Gluten free
Dairy free

Index

First published in the United Kingdom in 2013 by

Collins & Brown

10 Southcombe Street

London

W14 0RA

An imprint of Anova Books Company Ltd

Based on an original concept by Hearst Books, a division of Sterling Publishing Co., Inc., from
Good Housekeeping: DROP 5 LBS by Heather K. Jones., RD, edited by Rosemary Ellis, editor-in-chief Good Housekeeping

The Good Housekeeping website is
www.allboutyou.com/goodhousekeeping

10 9 8 7 6 5 4 3 2

ISBN 978-1-908449-15-3

A catalogue record for this book is available from the British Library.

Reproduction by Dot Gradations Ltd, UK
Printed and bound by GZ Printek, Spain
Illustrations by Beci Orpin

This book can be ordered direct from the publisher at
www.anovabooks.com

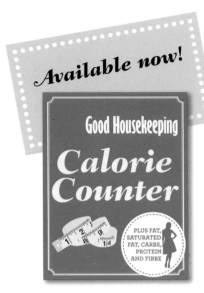

Available now!

Good Housekeeping

Calorie Counter

PLUS FAT, SATURATED FAT, CARBS, PROTEIN AND FIBRE

This book can be ordered direct from the publisher at www.anovabooks.com

£5.99 | ISBN 978-1-908449-26-9